Bart Willigers lives with his wife, two children, and a dog in Suffolk, England. In early 2022, Bart was diagnosed with a brain tumour. This diagnosis was a defining moment in Bart's life. It called for a change in priorities and lifestyle choices. Nevertheless, Bart continues to work as a decision analyst.

To Sandy, Anneke and Thomas

Bart Willigers

INSIGHT

How Decision Analysis Relieved a Life Crisis

AUSTIN MACAULEY PUBLISHERS™

LONDON * CAMBRIDGE * NEW YORK * SHARJAH

A CIP catalogue record for this title is available from the British Library.

ISBN 9781035840953 (Paperback)
ISBN 9781035840960 (Hardback)
ISBN 9781035840977 (ePub e-book)

www.austinmacauley.com

First Published 2024
Austin Macauley Publishers Ltd®
1 Canada Square
Canary Wharf
London
E14 5AA

My life has been a rollercoaster ever since the doctors found a golf ball-sized tumour in my brain. There are so many people who helped, were willing to listen, gave comfort, and lifted my spirits. I am grateful to all of you.

I am incredibly grateful to my wife, Sandy, and our children, Anneke and Thomas. The three of you mean everything to me.

My parents, Joke and Hans, my brother, Ton, my sister-in-law, Mirjam, my niece, and my nephew, made each trip back home to the Netherlands very special to me.

My mother-in-law, Margaret, and the Austin family for being so incredibly inviting and making me feel at home in the UK.

I am blessed with my family and friends. I am forever indebted by the support you have given me. The family and friends from the village in the Netherlands where I grew up, my university friends both in Utrecht and in Copenhagen, and the village friends in the two villages where I have lived since, I moved to the UK.

I especially would like to thank all my uncles, aunts, cousins, and nieces. My sincere appreciation to you all, your support has been second to none. I am forever grateful to all of you.

Marcel van Gaalen, Tanni Abramovitz, Tod Waight, Joel Baker, Armelle Kloppenburg, Marco van der Meulen, Rob van Eijs, Andor Lips, the Smart family, and all the local friends who support us daily and who drove me to the hospital for radiation treatment – five days a week for a six week's period.

I am indebted to my colleagues who have read many, many previous drafts of the manuscript. I would like to especially mention Mario Ouwens, David Wright, Dougan McKellar, Sridevi Nagarajan, Martin Simán, Patrick Darken, Ioannis

Psallidas, Stephen Baker, Névine Zariffa, Paul Metcalfe, Erik Hermansson, Bruce Potter, Sarah Vowler, Elisabeth Nyman, Chris Miller, Mishal Patel, Jim Weatherall, Eleanor Fung, Martin Jenkins, Karin Bowen, Ian Hirsch, Gabriella Rustici, Beth Duncan, and Anne Radcliff.

I would also like to acknowledge the Society of Decision Professionals for creating a community of likeminded individuals across the globe. I am particularly grateful to Larry Lawrence, Ralph Keeney, Pete Naylor, Babak Jafarizadeh, Wayne Borchardt, Blyth Warwick, Andrea Dickens, Johnnie Moore, Dave Levin, and David Spiegelhalter. I thank Reidar Bratvold, Stephen Begg, and Frank Koch for introducing me to the field of decision analysis.

I am very grateful to the medical team and all the nurses who looked after me during my illness. The care I received was second to none. Although it is easy to criticise the National Health Service (NHS) without the help of the medical team and nurses, I would not have been able to have finished this book.

Finally, I would like to thank Archie. Archie, who has taken me on many walks in the Suffolk countryside. Archie, you make me smile with every wag of your tail.

Table of Contents

Part 1

Synopsis

2022 was supposed to be the best year of my career. Being in my early 50s, I was about to complete my first decade working in the pharmaceutical industry. I would be lying if I said that the transition from the energy industry to pharmaceuticals was easy, but after a few difficult years, I felt confident about the future. Then one day, I was rushed to the hospital because I had collapsed in the garden. A scan showed that I had a brain tumour. From that day onwards, matters changed dramatically; things that were important to me before lost all their value, whilst other things that I had taken for granted before suddenly became very important to me.

This book is my attempt to make a difference for all people who are suffering from a terminal illness, or indeed all people who must make personal decisions at difficult and emotionally charged times. This book is intended for individuals who wish to improve their decision-making skills using structured and analytical thinking. In this personal book, I am using examples and thought experiments to illustrate how decision analysis can be used to increase our awareness of available choices and uncertainties.

Introduction

'This is your last chance. After this, there is no turning back. You take the blue pill – the story ends. You wake up in your bed and believe whatever you want to believe. You take the red pill – you stay in Wonderland and I show you how deep the rabbit hole is. Remember, all I'm offering are the truth. Nothing more.'

The Matrix, the first of a sequel of four feature films

Abstract Introduction

I believe that it is nearly impossible to think rationally about decisions when you have just discovered that your life has been shortened by several decades. I did not sleep in the summer of 2022. At least that is how it felt at the time. During the day, I was working on this book. At night, I was tossing and turning in bed. My wife told me that I was frequently snoring – so clearly, I got some sleep in those early days after the tumour had been found.

Decisions that involve a critical illness are, per definition, heavily emotionally charged. Patients rarely have the appropriate skills to deal with situations in which they suddenly find themselves. Typically, there is great anxiety about the consequences of the decisions that patients are forced to make. There is time pressure and often a set of conflicting objectives. The optimal choice is often unclear because of the large number of uncertainty patients are exposed to. A typical decision pertaining to a critical illness does not come nicely wrapped in a bow. These decisions are typically messy, very messy.

Although I envisioned patients to be the prime audience, the techniques described are completely generic and can be applied to any difficult decision situation, e.g., business decisions, finding a new job, moving house, selecting a holiday destination, choosing a school, retirement planning, and buying company shares.

This book introduces decision analysis. Decision analysis helps to provide structure to complex decisions, applies analytical thinking to problems, and creates a set of insights. Once these insights are obtained, making the actual decision is straightforward.

'My name is Bart and I have a brain tumour.'

'My name is Bart and I have a brain tumour.'

That sounds very much like the first line uttered by the leading character in the opening scene of a film. His fellow members of Alcoholics Anonymous are sitting in a circle around him. A woman is fiddling with her hair, a man rubbing his feet on his chair, and another quickly looking up at the main character while he is speaking. However, this is not a fictional story; my tumour is real.

One month earlier, my life was very different. I was 51 years old and happily married to a caring wife with two lovely children. Living in the Suffolk countryside, southern England. I am Dutch but have lived most of my adult life abroad – Denmark, Germany, Scotland, and the past five years in England. I have a busy life with typical worries about ageing parents and all the well-known challenges of two growing teenagers. Our eldest started university last year, while our youngest is still living at home. My parents back in the Netherlands had their share of recent health issues – both being hospitalised in the past year.

However, there was also a perspective of a cancer-free future. My wife and I are both in our early 50s and reasonably fit; hence, I viewed the risk of being affected by cancer to be much lower than would warrant any worries. I considered the prospect of getting cancer as just of a larger set of issues that can affect all of us – 1 day. Therefore, in the spring of 2022, in the post-COVID-19 lockdown era, we started the discussion on how to make the most of the upcoming summer.

Professionally, things were looking good too! After the 2015–2016 collapse of oil prices, I faced the prospect of redundancy. Fortunately, one of the large pharmaceutical companies threw me a lifeline. I joined my current employer in the fall of 2016. Admittedly, I had a rough start. The corporate culture was very different, with a change in industry and ever-changing priorities from management. However, professional things fell into place in 2021, and I was feeling confident that 2022 would be my best year yet.

The 20th of March 2022 was the day that everything changed. On that day, I was rushed to the hospital after I collapsed in the garden. I was told I had a "suspected seizure". I knew that the probability of something serious was very small; therefore, at the time, I was convinced that the CT scan would not show anything.

How wrong I was. A CT scan showed that I had a brain tumour. That single image of my brain changed my life forever.

On 8th May 2022, I wrote a letter to my mother-in-law. Much had happened in the period that had passed since I last saw her in early April. In the letter, I explained to her how my value system had changed – things that were important to me before lost all their value, while other things that I had taken for granted before suddenly became essential to me. My notion of time also changed. Time had suddenly become very precious to me. I also told her that I felt physically and mentally completely fine. I was expecting that this would change once I started my treatment.

In my letter, I told my mother-in-law that I was determined to make more time for my family and that I wanted to ensure that I had told the children all that I wanted to tell them. I started writing a diary and an autobiography in parallel[1]. With the eldest child studying philosophy and psychology and the youngest child who never voluntarily entered a library, I understood that I was facing a tough crowd.

Once I finished writing the letter, I felt a strange sense of guilt. I felt so normal. I started the day by reading a book about Napoleon written by the Flemish writer Bart van Loo. I spend 40–50 minutes reading about his crossing of the Mediterranean back to France after his escape to Egypt. After breakfast, the three of us, my wife, our youngest child, and I, went to check out some garden furniture in Sudbury. After lunch, I joined my village friends to drink a couple of beers.

I questioned my sanity. How could I feel so normal just 12 days after a brain CT scan triggered a personal judgement that my life had been shortened by 24 years? I pinched my arm to ensure that I was fully conscious.

To this day, I struggle to get my head around this – I had a brain tumour the size of a golf ball in my head, and I simply did not notice it at all. Utterly bizarre!

That evening, I sat down to watch the late BBC evening news. I poured myself a Belgium Trappist beer. Obviously, using an original Trappist glass. I

---

[1] At this stage, I had not conceived the idea of writing a book for terminally ill patients and their carers. Over time, it dawned on me that the methods were sufficiently generic that they could be useful to all people facing tough decisions.

drank half of it. I poured the remainder down the sink. That was the first Belgium Trappist beer I had thrown away.

Introduction to Decision Analysis

The origin of the word "decide" is the Latin word "decider", meaning "to cut off" as in slicing away alternatives. A frequently quoted statistic is that people make 35,000 decisions each day[2]. This equates to one decision every 2.5 seconds.

Before deciding, you must be aware that there is a decision to be made. A decision starts with a thought. One study estimated that humans have approximately 6,000 thoughts per day using functional magnetic resonance imaging (fMRI)[3]. Six thousand daily thoughts is a large number but significantly less than the 35,000 decisions quoted before. Part of the difference might be explained by the fact that the human mind is unconsciously aware of most decisions humans make. Most decisions to keep the human body functioning are made subconsciously. This is presumably done to free up our cognitive abilities for more important thoughts. Although we all have the impression that we can make our own choices, this subjective experience of freedom is no more than an illusion.

Only a small proportion of these 6,000 thoughts will be related to decisions, and most of these decisions are trivial, e.g., will you drink your coffee black or with a splash of milk? But some of them are truly important, such as what activities are you pursuing during your final year of life? Should you participate in this clinical trial?[4] The focus of this book is on the latter type of decisions. Those that require careful thought and structure. Decisions are conscious acts. You must allocate effort to define your personal values, identify your decisions and choices, and the consequences associated with these choices.

I cannot overstress the importance of following good decision-making practises. Choosing wisely is a life skill[5]. Most of us have not been formally trained in decision making. Decision analysis is a discipline used to transform opaque decision problems into a transparent sequence of steps. Decision analysis

---

[2] https://go.roberts.edu/leadingedge/the-great-choices-of-strategic-leaders

[3] Tseng and Poppenk, 2020.

[4] Much more mundane decisions relate to whether you should accept a job offer, move house, which car to buy, and where to go on holiday.

[5] Believe me, the irony of calling it a life skill, given that I am terminally ill and that a high percentage of my intended readership would also be, is not lost on me.

offers the creation of clear insight that provides guidance on which course of action is preferred.

Although the ultimate outcome of a situation is beyond your influence, you can increase the chance of a desired outcome by maximising the quality of your decisions. "Quality" means making a decision that leads to a favourable outcome.

Here is a quick example. Imagine that you and your partner went out for dinner at a fancy restaurant. You ordered some champagne and a bottle of red wine to celebrate your fifth wedding anniversary. After dessert, you asked for the bill and ordered a taxi home. On the way home, the taxi driver had an accident, and your partner was severely injured.

The fact that your partner was injured is just bad luck, a bad break. The decision you made to order the taxi was a good decision. The quality of the decision was good at the time and will remain good forever (Figure 1.1).

Now imagine a second scenario. Again, you and your partner sat down for dinner and had a few drinks. This time around, you grabbed the car keys home drove home yourself. 30 minutes later, you safely parked the car in the garage. Poor decision but good outcome. This latter situation is sometimes referred to as "dumb luck".

To reiterate, the quality of a decision can only be judged by the knowledge available at the time the decision was made, the logic applied to arrive at the decision, our value system (objectives), and the alternatives. A good outcome is simply a desirable state of the world.

Outcome

		Good	Bad
Quality of decision	Good	Deserved Success	Bad Break
	Bad	Dumb Luck	Justice

Figure 1.1. Quality of decision versus outcome.

After the decision has been made, you cannot change the quality of that decision and must leave the rest to chance, but you can certainly stack the cards in your favour! Good decision making will improve the likelihood of achieving a desired outcome. You can assess the quality of your decision at the time of your decision by answering a set of very basic questions. These questions act as a checklist for each of the six decision elements:

What is the scope of the decision (Frame);
What is the objective of the decision maker (Values);
What are the available alternatives (Alternatives);
What information is available and is it reliable? (Information);
Can you articulate why you have chosen your preferred option? (Reasoning);
Are you fully committed to your decision? (Commitment to action).

These questions are referred to as Decision Quality[6].

Decision analysis is a social activity. Decision analysis tools are communication aids that can be used to create insight into the decisions you face. There are many decision analysis tools, not all of which are useful or practical when coping with a terminal illness. In this situation, you are not seeking to maximise profit, minimise timelines or minimise costs. Rather, you interested in creating insights around the uncertainties you are faced with and identifying the decisions that are available to you. Decision analysis uses visual images to tell a story using clear, simple language and logic that is nevertheless specific and articulate.

Let me repeat. The objective of decision analysis is to create insight that provides clarity on what to do next. There are situations that require continuous updating of your decision model. However, one can stop the analysis if further analysis does not alter the choice, you are about to make. Humans tend to search through the available alternatives until an acceptable threshold is met. This cognitive heuristic is referred to as "satisficing"[7].

---

[6] More information on Decision Quality is provided later in this book.
[7] Simon, 1945.

Imagine that you are invited for a fancy lunch. One might be tempted to overfill one's plate just with the starters[8]. However, in the decision analysis approach, you would first review the entire menu: from the dessert to the main course and finally to the starters. Only after you have established what the full menu involves would you dig in. Making the right choices is a key component of good decision making.

I should mention that I have been a decision analyst for the past twenty years and played various roles in pharmaceutical companies and in the energy sector. In this capacity, I have helped many experts enhance their judgements on survival rates, improve assessments of trade-offs, and quantify economic benefits. The truth is that the ability to make good decisions is not inborn. Even though the fact that we survived as a species suggests that the decisions our predecessors made were "good enough", some people might still argue that the ability to make good decisions is contrary to human nature[9].

Over the years, I have come to realise that difficult decisions involve the following:

1) a very large degree of uncertainty, or;
2) trade-offs between incompatible values (e.g., Quality of Life versus cost).

These two types of problems are explored in this book.

I will draw upon each of the two competing philosophies in decision analysis: management science and psychology. Management science talks about how we should make decisions and is all about achieving an objective, that is, maximising an objective function. It identifies the optimal decisions given the information, alternatives, and preferences. Psychology describes how the human mind makes a judgement and how this judgement is used to make decisions. Psychology uses insights from behavioural studies that discuss biases that result from rule-of-thumb (heuristics) decisions and point to inconsistencies and illogical thinking. These thinking errors are the root cause of the poor decisions that humans make. We continually reach undesirable outcomes because of suboptimal, even poor, decisions.

---

[8] 'Appetizers' is the American equivalent to 'starters'.
[9] Spetzler et al., 2016.

In my opinion, both philosophies can bring about insights, which is the goal of decision analysis.

The term *"decision analysis"* was coined by Ronald Howard in the 1980s. When Howard was asked in 2011 about the challenge of decision analysis, he replied, 'The willingness to employ [decision analysis].' I have spent many years wondering why decision analysis has not gained wider acceptance. I believe that this lack of acceptance is related to biases in our thinking. The way we perceive the world is a simplified version of reality. Our brain creates a coherent version of the world in which we live. It is difficult, or even impossible, to see beyond these biases, even if you know you are being tricked[10]. People widely believe that they are inherently good decision makers, but this belief is an illusion – a dangerous one[11].

A second reason that decision analysis has not caught on is that it requires practise. People need time to master the skills required to be an effective decision maker. We are so busy. Simply coping and dealing with life takes up all our time and energy. Most of the studies on decision analysis focus on business problems, typical examples of which include cash flow calculations structured in decision trees and project prioritisation exercises. The problem with these decisions is that the project timelines of these business problems are simply too long; therefore, people involved in these projects cannot practise their decision-making skills. For example, it takes many years to run a clinical trial; therefore, employees cannot develop their decision-making skills.

Personal decision making is different. There are numerous personal decisions that you must make during your life. Hence, there is plenty of scope for practise. Also, these decisions are highly relevant to you personally, particularly if you have been recently diagnosed with a terminal illness. These decisions are also simple in the sense that you, the patient, are in charge. Although the impact might extend to your family and close friends, you are the main person affected. There are no politics.

A third reason is that in the post-COVID-19 pandemic world, data have taken the central stage. Although I can see a large overlap between the Decision Quality process and the PPDAC[12] cycle. The PPDAC cycle is the approach

---

[10] I will show you an example in one of the following chapters that will hopefully convince you.

[11] Spetzler et al., 2016.

[12] PPDAC is an abbreviation for problem, plan, data, analysis, conclusion.

advocated by statisticians and data scientists to conduct statistical investigations. The cycle that is used consists of five stages: problem, plan, data, analysis, and conclusion. However, an increasing number of people want to make "data-driven decisions", and the absence of a *decision* seems like a notable omission. It appears to me that no value is created if you do not act on the insight you have developed.

Finally, I do subscribe to the view expressed by members of the communities of statisticians and data scientists that the lack of basic knowledge of mathematics and statistics is one of the core challenges of this century. The ability to investigate a dataset using basic plots should be a skill that each school child should develop. The way statistics is taught at school has completely changed recently. A few decades ago, statistics was a rather dull topic about probability distributions and hypothesis testing. Nowadays, it is much more practical, and the focus is on problem solving. I wish I could make a similar contribution in the field of decision analysis; teach people the skills to enable them to make better decisions.

No one has chosen to become a patient with a terminal disease. In the end, it is very unfortunate to find yourself in a situation where you have terminal illness. This book is not intended for all patients with terminal illness. As a professional decision scientist, I understand that the methods described in this book will resonate only with a minority of terminally ill patients.

I suspect that few doctors choose medicine because of their interest in psychology and statistics. Nevertheless, I hope that this text can be used to connect with patients under their care. For patients who are willing to engage in decision analysis, I hope that the text provides guidance on how to structure their thinking.

On the importance of decision tools

As in any book, some parts are more important than others. I used a waterfall chart to assign a value to the various topics explained in this book (Figure 1.2). If nothing else, ensure that you understand the concepts described in the chapters *on Decision Analysis, Creativity*, and *Values.*

The chapter *Decision Analysis* describes the tools used to analyse your personal situation. *Decision Quality* is the tool that has the greatest potential. The

---

https://nzmaths.co.nz/category/glossary/statistical-enquiry-cycle

power of Decision Quality lies in its simplicity and general applicability; this method can be applied to all decisions. Adhering to the principles of this framework ensures that all decisions you make from today onward are of high quality. Decision Quality is instrumental in making better real-life decisions. Decision Quality is fundamentally different from the seemingly endless collection of 2 by 2 matrices with catchy acronyms such as SWOT, CATWOE, MoSCoW, or MOST. I called out these tools because I used to really dislike them whilst I was doing my MBA degree several decades ago; at the time, I considered them to be pointless[13].

The development of a correct *Frame* ensures that the analysis you are about to undertake is focussed on the correct problem. Frame is the starting point of the analysis. Hence, if an error is made in the frame, all the analyses that follow are at risk of being wasted effort. We need to be confident to get the frame right. The importance of the frame is illustrated by the fact that it is the first element of Decision Quality. Developing a frame typically involves writing a well-defined problem statement. It will take time and effort to develop such a problem statement, but it will pay off in the end. *Influence Diagram* is a very suitable communication method for collecting input from a group of stakeholders. Doctors, patients, and carers can all contribute by calling out concerns, considerations, or problems. These issues can be captured in a basic spreadsheet or displayed in a diagram. *Multi-Criteria Decision Analysis* (*MCDA*) is a technique that can be applied when a high degree of rigour is required. It is an algorithm based on double-relative ranking of 1) decision criteria and 2) alternatives. As the ranking is done on a relative basis, it caters to the strength of humans, i.e., it is much easier to make a relative judgement than an absolute judgement. For example, I found it easy to get to the topics in the correct order in Figure 1.2 using relative judgements.

The second most important, in my opinion, might seem a surprising choice as it relates to *Creativity*. Creativity is essential for developing various compelling objectives, choices, and consequences. Without creativity, it is simply impossible to develop a rich set of these three-fold issues. The approaches described will stimulate your creative thinking.

Values describes a methodology that can be used to define your personal objectives – what is your purpose in life? What makes you get up in the morning?

---

[13] Admittedly, over the years, the approach of putting succinct words in boxes has grown on me…

What makes you tick? Without having a crystal-clear understanding of what is truly important to you personally, you cannot make difficult decisions. I have dedicated an entire chapter to how to find your core values using Objective Networks. This chapter is heavily influenced by the book *Value-Focused Thinking* by Ralph Keeney14. Keeney makes the valid argument that you cannot decide what to choose if you do not know what you would like to achieve. There is rarely sufficient time and effort allocated to define one's personal objectives.

Human judgement describes an approach that minimises the impact of biases on our judgement through careful crafting of the questions we are answering. One of the key findings of recent psychological research is that our mind has a very limited awareness of what is going on around us. Our view of our environment is a simplified version of reality and is biased by our emotions and physical needs[15].

In my judgement, once you read and understood these four chapters, you are over 55% on your way to become a better decision-maker (Figure 1.2).

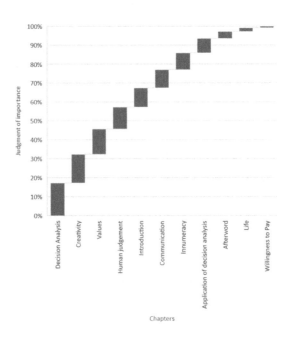

Figure 1.2. My personal judgement on the importance of the chapters in this book.

---

[14] Keeney, 1992.

[15] E.g., hunger and sexual drive.

Concluding remarks: Introduction

After I saw the image of my brain tumour, I decided to start writing a diary. Parts of the diary eventually became part of this book. Soon after I started my diary, I also started writing an autobiography. I wanted to tell our children the story of my life – I was really determined to finish my autobiography before Christmas 2022. In the autumn of 2022, I began writing this book on decision analysis and my illness. At the time, I was not sure whether my life was long enough to complete it.

During this period, I have made many decisions that are of great importance to me. I have analysed what to do with, what I felt at the time, the final months of my life. Decision analysis is my coping mechanism. I am a "number guy" and by developing frameworks and analysing numbers, I created the insights I needed to make the right choices.

Writing this book has been a personal journey and, as time was literally of the essence, I was forced to make continuous trade-offs and set priorities on what chapter to tackle next. Part of the process was to define small targets that I was confident I could manage.

I am very grateful that I can share the knowledge that I have accumulated over the past 20 years with you.

Although there are a significant number of statistical topics described in this book, I would like to stress that much of the benefit of decision analysis can be realised without having any knowledge about statistics. Much of the value that decision analysis offers can be realised by being clear and effective in communication with stakeholders, being creative, having a well-defined values system and by developing a clearly defined problem that requires analysis.

The book has four parts. You have reached the end of the first part. The second part describes the recent events that shaped my life and the decisions I had to make during that period. The second part concludes with reflections on my life and death. The third part provides a description of the different approaches and methods I have used to ensure that I made the optimal choice in each situation. The fourth part concludes the book with some final thoughts.

Part 2

Surviving

'Our unconscious therefore does not believe in its own death; it acts as though it were immortal.'

Sigmund Freud in *Reflections on War and Death*

'The word hope first appeared in English about a thousand years ago, denoting a combinations of confidence and desire. But what I desired – life – was not what I was confident about – death... When I talked about hope, then, did I really mean "Leave some room for a statistically improbable but still plausible outcome – a survival just above the measured 95% confidence interval?" Is that what hope was? Could we divide the curve into existential sections, from "defeated" to "pessimistic" to "realistic" to "hopeful" to "delusional"? Had we all just given in to the "hope" that every patient was above average?'

Paul Kalanithi in *When Breath Becomes Air*

Abstract Surviving

My collapse in the garden triggered a chain of events that eventually led to the diagnosis of a brain tumour. On the 26th of April 2022, I was confronted with my own mortality for the first time.

I am employed as a decision analyst for a pharmaceutical company. As a decision analyst, it is my job to ensure that the best possible decisions are consistently made. Over the past decades, I have compiled a comprehensive toolkit. The tools were specifically chosen to analyse a very broad range of decisions, and all the tools serve to create the largest number of insights using the least amount of effort. All the tools I applied to my personal situation are very practical – I did not want to waste any time on any of the decisions I have made over the past two years!

However, I am also a mortal human being. I am an individual who has contracted a terminal illness – I am a patient. The realisation that I am a mortal being made me hyperaware of my value system. Also, I had a strong desire to make the best possible decisions, communicate the expected progression of my illness as best as I possibly could, make a judgement on the length of my remaining life (Overall Survival) that was both accurate and precise, and make a thorough re-assessment on the remaining life span as I underwent a series of MRI scans, surgical, pharmacological, and radiotherapies.

I have contemplated, analysed, what to do with the final part of my life. Some decisions were easy. For example, I had to go back to work in September 2022. Life without work would have driven me insane. Therefore, no analysis was required for that decision. Other decisions were more complex and required the development of a structure, and some decisions needed a decision model.

What follows is a chronological series of events that have shaped my life during the past year and a bit…

My decision diary

20 March 2022: I collapsed in the garden

BBC Headline: With 37 million in lockdown and Covid plans under fire, Chinese ask: what comes next?

The account of the collapse

The epilepsy nurse made the following statement:
'This morning I met Bart and his wife. Bart can recall going on a bike ride on Sunday of around 60 km. He then came home and had lunch and then went out with his son to trim the hedge. He says that he felt quite strange whilst doing it and felt like it was harder than normal. The next thing he remembers is lying on the ground with his wife next to him, saying "Squeeze my hand". He recalls the arrival of the ambulance.

Bart's son says that he was not watching Bart; however, he noticed that the hedge clippers stopped and went to investigate and found Bart lying face down and the hedge clipper cutters a couple of metres away. Bart's wife remarks that her son felt that he looked like he was dead. Bart's son then shouted for his Mum, who was on the other side of the hedge, and when she arrived, Bart was faced down. She rolled him over to determine what had happened. She thought he had cut himself. His arms were moving like he was trying to get off his gloves. He was not stiff or floppy; his eyes were open and fixed; when he came around, he was very confused and started walking everywhere. Gradually, over 5 or 10 minutes, he started getting back to responding and chatting, and then after 20 minutes, he was back to his normal self.

Bart did not bite his tongue nor was he incontinent of urine, and when he was in the ambulance, he said that he did not feel tired nor did his body ache.

Bart stated that he felt that he might have been dehydrated as he did not drink any water after the bike ride, whereas usually, he would drink around 3 glasses of water. He has been sleeping well and is quite stressed at work. He works for a pharmaceutical company.

When arriving in the emergency department, his ECG was completed with a QTc of 435, his blood sugar was 6.4, and a CT head was not performed at the time.'

This story was recorded by the epilepsy nurse on the 28th of March 2022.

System 1 thinking: stick to the base rate

After my collapse in our garden, I convinced myself that I had simply fainted. The combination of a long bike ride in the morning, followed by a quick lunch with not sufficient to drink and the hard labour of hedge cutting in the afternoon made up a plausible story. I created a plausible story to satisfy System 1 thinking. Using System 1, I dismissed the facts that 1) "His arms were moving like he was trying to get off his gloves", 2) "He was very confused and getting up to walk everywhere", 3) "Gradually over 5 or 10 minutes he started getting back to responding".

I also did not expect that the tests scheduled for me would find anything. I had little faith in the cardio activity monitoring and CT scan that the doctors had scheduled on my behalf. I was feeling healthy, and I kept telling myself, 'There is nothing wrong with you.'

Given that I simply did not expect that the tests would show anything, I stuck with the base rate. In my judgement, there was a very low probability that I was seriously ill. Also, if any tests showed something that would be so bad, I was not willing to engage in that line of thinking.

I was also affected by motivational bias. I was most concerned about losing my driving license 6 months without a driving licence seemed like a very long time. I had a strong alternative motive to simply assume that I was healthy.

System 1 thinking is a way of thinking that comes naturally to us. System 1 thinking requires little effort and is our default way of perceiving the world around us. My system 1 drew conclusions that simplified reality by placing more emphasis on the fact that I felt healthy at the time and ignored some of the facts raised by the nurse. I did not want to engage in a line of thought that something was seriously wrong with me. It was altogether easier to stick with the base rate: I was active and reasonably fit in my early 50s.

25 April 2022: CT scan

The CT scanner was placed in a container in a parking lot at the back of West Suffolk Hospital. My wife dropped me off, and I waited next to the container to be invited to enter the scanner.

Back home, I noticed that the soles of my 20-year old shoes had perished.

26 April 2022: Tumour found and the need for high-quality decisions

BBC Headline: The world's richest man Elon Musk acquires Twitter in a 44 billion dollar deal

I was interrupted by my wife during a conference call. The hospital phoned to ask whether we could have a meeting that same afternoon. I was worried. The severity of the situation was confirmed in the hospital when we were told that the consultant had not signed in for the afternoon.

We were told that an abnormality was to be observed on the CT scan of my brain. There appeared to be a tumour in the left frontal lobe with a fair amount of swelling. The swelling around the tumour could indicate rapid growth of the tumour. To reduce the swelling in my brain, I immediately started steroid treatment.

On our way back from the hospital, we laid down one ground rule. This illness should not define us. No one is helped by sitting around the kitchen table feeling sorry for each other.

We also decided to sell a car, update, and collect pension information, and plan how to tell the children, my parents, and my brother. Four decisions made during a 30-min drive back home from the hospital!

Once we returned from the hospital, my thoughts turned to a framework that I have frequently applied during the last twenty years of my career: Decision Quality. In this period, I have taught this framework to literally hundreds, if not thousands, of professionals in both the pharmaceutical and energy sectors. I received emails out of the blue from people I had only the faintest recollection of thanking for sharing this single piece of advice.

The key benefits of this method are its simplicity and general applicability; any decision can be analysed using this framework. Decision Quality states that all decisions have six elements. Not four or five, but precisely six elements are required to define a valid decision. The reason for having six elements is that you cannot make a high-quality decision if any or multiple elements are not explicitly addressed. Figure 2.1 shows the elements as a chain. This chain is a reference to the weakest link. A decision is only as good as the weakest link in the chain. Use the remaining time on the element that has the lowest perceived score.

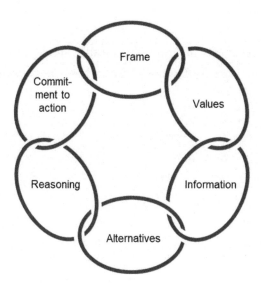

Figure 2.1. The six elements of decision quality. The diagram is shown as a chain because it symbolises the weakest link, the weakest link on which you must focus your effort.

A decision implies the existence of

1. Frame: Scope of the decision
2. Values: The objective the decision-maker is trying to maximise or minimise
3. Alternatives: Multiple alternatives must exist to enable the decision maker to make a choice.
4. Information: In the absence of information, a decision maker will be indifferent to alternatives
5. Reasoning: A decision maker must be able to articulate his or her preferences
6. Commitment to action: Contemplating different choices is fundamentally different from making a commitment to take forward an alternative

This framework, these six elements, can be applied to all decisions. This framework was holding the key to not losing my sanity on this fateful day – the 26th of April 2022.

Email to my consultant

Reflecting on the events that unfolded on that Sunday, I realised that I was biased. I am very grateful to the consultant whose judgement was much less biased than mine. I wrote her an email:

Dear consultant,

I would like you to know that my wife and I are very grateful for your swift actions after reviewing my CT scan.

An operation is scheduled for May 25.

Although I am fully aware of the long way that lies ahead, for certain, you have increased my probability of long-term survival!

Kindest regards,
Bart Willigers

The last sentence of the message was a reference to my insistence during our last conversation to obtain some probabilistic input to several scenarios I created.

At the time, I was told that she did not feel qualified to give me these probabilities. She told me 'You are not a statistic!' I fundamentally disagree with that statement; I am a decision analyst after all.

The last sentence contained a small joke. In the third paragraph, I added "for certain". In my assessment, there was a 55% probability that she would pick up on this.

29 April 2022: Society of Decision Professionals

In the afternoon, I went for my usual Friday afternoon bike ride. As a safety precaution, I invited a friend from the village to join me so that he could call for assistance if I did get another seizure. I admittedly did not tell him this. I had one seizure over a month ago, so the probability of a second occurrence during a 90-min interval was assessed as an acceptable risk. This was our first ride together, and after I cycled to the top of the hill just outside our village, I seemed to have lost my friend. I waited for my friend to arrive. I sent a route description to him in the morning, so I was reasonably confident that we could continue our bike ride. We lost each other during the final part of the ride. I had to rush back to my next conference call.

While I was dressing myself after my shower, my consultant called to check up on me. I told her that I followed the advice on not searching the internet for "growing brain tumours". I did not mention my bike ride. After 15 minutes, we ended the conversation, and I realised that I was getting cold as my upper body was bare, still drying after my shower.

In the evening, I was attending the annual conference of the Society of Decision Professionals. The Society of Decision Professionals has a global mission to enhance the quality of decisions. This was the second time I attended a US-based conference. I chaired a session on the Probability of Success. Probability of Success is the chance of a successful outcome, i.e., the chance that a well will produce oil or that a clinical trial is successful. Different industries face similar challenges. After the presentations, I led a question-and-answer session. The intent was to highlight how similar the challenges were across different industries. Afterwards, we entered a breakout room that remained open for another 45 min - a new record!

3 May 2022: Early in the morning

I hardly slept last night. I am suffering from side effects of my steroid treatment. My wife moved to a different bed during the night. At 5am, I switched off my usual 6:42 am alarm call…for ever? At 7:00 am, I heard the bath running and our son's music. I remained in bed until he finished his bath. Once I heard him opening the bathroom door, I got up and stepped into the shower.

4 May 2022: The first MRI scan

BBC Headline: EU proposes a total ban on Russian oil imports

Today, I have a 13:00 appointment for an MRI scan. After my wife dropped me off at the hospital entrance, I made my way to the MRI department. I was surprised at how familiar this small hospital in Bury St Edmunds, Suffolk, feels after just two visits in a little over a month. At this time, the COVID-19 restrictions in public spaces have been completely lifted, except in hospitals. I navigated the hospital as an early morning commuter found his way through a busy railway station. I noticed an elderly man with a walking stick, a young doctor rushing past me, and a mother trying to console her young daughter. Upon entering the MRI department, I heard a sound unfamiliar to me. The sound came from an MRI machine that was working. Once the required forms were completed and I changed into a blue gown, I was taken to the MRI room and laid down on a bench ready for my scan.

The sound inside the machine is deafening. I felt the bench moving forward and backward while my brain was sliced into a series of scans. I could faintly hear the 1980s band Roxette. While the MRI machine was violently shaking and humming, I was reminded of the lyric "C'mon join the joyride".

Walking back to the hospital exit, I felt positive. Gradually, my mood dampened somewhat as I became very aware of the fact that these are still early days in my illness. I simply did not know how the known-unknowns and unknown-unknowns – to use Donald Rumsfeld's categorisation of uncertainties – will present itself and how these would affect me and my close family. I felt blissfully ignorant!

6 May 2022: Learning about my illness

I woke up early today. I could still feel the area of shorter hair on my chest where the ambulance staff cleared a small area to stick the plaster. Connected to this plaster were the wires that were wired into a machine that measured my cardiac function. It felt like a long time ago – the day I was rushed to the hospital after my "first suspected seizure".

I planned to tell my colleagues about my illness. I had already arranged for an hour call with a colleague who is very dear to me. We have been collaborating for years. Unfortunately, we had fallen out around the time our project was finally presented to the company board. I felt really bad about the way I had treated her. We had a great conversation, and we talked about the next projects that we should be working on! She also insisted that I should not waste any time and try to get support from colleagues. She listed a couple of colleagues with oncology backgrounds – one of whom I knew. I arranged a call with that colleague and me wife the same afternoon.

The next 30 min, I wrote several meeting requests with the general message "I need to tell you something personal." One colleague replied via an instant message: 'nothing seriously I hope?' I replied '…I have a brain tumour…'

I had three other short work phone calls before our meeting with a colleague that was very knowledgeable about oncology. The three of us spoke for 40 minutes. During this call, I received the first scientific facts on the factors that impact survival in brain oncology.

After ending the call, I jumped straight onto the next call with my sister-in-law. In the morning, I had sent her a message that I wanted to talk to that afternoon. She was aware of my suspected seizure. I realised that she would have taken the hint. The objective of this call was to plan on how to tell my parents. My parents were on their way home from southern France. Dad was in great pain and needed a doctor. In addition, one of my mother's sisters was about to start her treatment for breast cancer[16]. Overall, a tricky situation that required careful messaging on the details of my illness.

My wife and I discussed how to tell our children.

Later in the afternoon, whilst cutting the lawn, I realised that whatever was happening next, this illness would have a defining impact on me and my family.

---

[16] This year, two of Mum's sisters had been diagnosed with cancer. One with breast cancer and the second with pancreatic cancer.

7 May 2022: Elicitation before biopsy results

BBC Headline: Does the US really have the world's highest Covid death toll?

In the first week of May 2022, I made my first judgement of how much time I had left. I estimated that I had more than a 10% chance to survive the next 5 months and less than 10% to live another 30 years. I estimated my medium overall survival at 6 years. In my judgement, I was equally likely to die before or after six years of a brain tumour.

I did not mention this assessment to my consultant because I did not want to trigger a seizure in her brain. The advice she gave me was, 'Try not to worry,' which is not a great piece of advice for someone who is an expert in the development of judgements[17]!

The probabilistic assessment reflects my personal knowledge of the situation. I listened to my consultant and did not search for "brain tumour" online. I sat down and reflected deeply on the knowledge I had. I knew one person who died of a brain tumour. My father-in-law was fixing his roof at the end of October, and he was cremated the following March. The disease had progressed too far for treatment by the time he was diagnosed. The diagnosis came too late[18]. I got a real shock when I saw him around Christmas. He was deteriorating very quickly. He was sleeping more and more until 1 day he did not wake up. I would be surprised if my decline was faster than his. I was pretty confident that my decline would take longer, so I assigned a P10 of 5 months. I was 90% confident that I would still be alive during the first week of November.

My Dad turned 80 this year. I was 90% confident that I would not reach the grand age of 80. I assumed that that scenario was unlikely to happen. One must be careful that motivational biases are properly accounted for; I really want to reach an average life span of 81 years for males.

Finally, I estimated P50, also known as median or 50th percentile. The P50 splits the probability distribution in half, i.e., you are indifferent whether the true value is higher or lower than the P50. I only assessed P50 after I had carefully considered the extreme values, P10 and P90. I was sitting somewhere between

---

[17] Admittedly, my judgement was off by 4.5 years. I had severely underestimated the severity of my illness.

[18] As it turned out, both my father-in-law and I suffered from glioblastoma. The probability of that happening is very small. With an incidence of 3.21 per 100,000 makes a probability that the two of us suffer from the same illness about 0.00000000103…

my Dad and my father-in-law. Both men had suffered from cancer. My Dad had been diagnosed with prostate cancer, and I knew that prostate cancer can be treated very effectively if diagnosed early. I also knew that brain cancer is a very serious illness. I was not sure, at the time, whether the tumour was cancerous or benign. There were some indications that indicated a fast-growing tumour. There was a sign of swelling surrounding the tumour visible on the scans. Swellings are generally associated with fast-growing tumours.

Ultimately, I decided on my P50 to be six years. The results show that two scans made of my brain had reduced my expected life span by 25 years.

The probability distribution as defined by P10, P50, and P90 is very flat. Uncertainties with a flat distribution are characterised by a large variability, i.e., the uncertain variable can take several values. Such flat probability distributions are not very informative. We simply lack high-quality information that makes one part of the distribution more probable than the remainder of the distribution.

In my judgement, the probability distribution was also highly skewed. The difference between P10 and P50 is much smaller than the difference between P50 and P90[19].

My consultant told me that one of the side effects of taking a large daily dose of steroids is insomnia. After I started taking steroids, I started to wake up very early on most days. This might sound crazy and absurd, but I actually enjoy these early mornings. Our village is very quiet. After we moved into our house nearly six years ago, all four of us were a little surprised on our first morning that we had not heard a single human-made sound all night. This morning, I woke up around 3:30. For the first hour, there was not a single sound. Between 4:30 and 5:15, the birds woke up and gradually the volume of the bird noise increased.

---

[19] There is a 50% chance that the value lies between 0 and 6 years, and there is a 50% chance that the value exceeds 6 years. Using 122 years as an upper bound, we can assess the probability for the two regions using two uniform distributions, i.e., a flat distribution where each value has the same probability. The uniform distribution corresponding to the lower segment is 8.3% (50%/6 years = 8.33 %/year), and the uniform distribution corresponding to the upper segment is 0.43%. The probability density in the lower segment, values between 0 and 6 years, is about 20 times higher than that of the higher segment, values between 6 and 122 years. (Per definition, 40% of the possible values fall between the P10 and P50and another 40% of possible values between the P50 and P90. 40%/(6-(5/12)) years = 7.16 %/year; 40%/(80-6) years = 0.54 %/year; 7.16/0.54 = 13.25. Although this value is smaller than 20, it is still much higher in the lower half than in the upper half.)

Sunrise at 5:15. At that time, bird noise decreased and the sounds of the sheep in the paddock next to our house dominated.

Apart from the first suspected seizure, which I now suspect was an actual seizure, on the 20th of March, I feel no different than a year ago. No headaches, no signs of memory loss (my wife might not agree on this…) and hardly an increased sensation of tiredness. For now, I feel absolutely fine. During these early mornings, I have a very clear head to think about what to do with the remaining time. Time has suddenly become very precious.

My steroid prescription was given for a month. I hope my clear head holds up until my prescription runs out.

Different qualities of the data

The three-point estimates I developed gave me a strange sense of ease whilst waiting for the news from the hospital. At the time, I had very little information. This lack of data prevented me from making a precise judgement. I was waiting for the biopsy results, which I would only get after my surgery. The biopsy results are what I would refer to as "very high-quality" data – data that would dramatically affect one's judgement. Although biopsy results yield very high-quality data, the information is still not perfect. Like all tests, biopsy results have limitations. The degree of aggressiveness of the tumour is measured as the speed of cell division. The speed of cell division must be measured and extrapolated to the real world of my brain. Errors will be made in this extrapolation calculation, i.e., some degree of ambiguity persists.

MRI scans yield "high-quality" data. The images created by MRI scans are of high resolution, but the resolution is not of the quality that can be used to rule out the presence of cancer cells. The fact that there is no visible sign of cancer cells does not mean that there are none.

The most difficult data type to deal with is "current health" – how much energy do you have? Any pains? Seizures? The reason why dealing with these data is so bloody hard is that these data play havoc with the placebo effect and biases. Once a doctor prompts you if you are in any pain, placebo and biases kick in and it is very hard to reply unbiased.

8 May 2022: Coping with practical issues

We had friends over for dinner. Dinner and form-signing. As a Dutch individual form-signing is a strange activity. Basically, what is the point of getting a person to sign of form stating that you are known by this person and that you are fully cognitively functioning? Maybe it is the same in the Netherlands, I have never lived in the Netherlands with a terminal illness.

It takes a lot of effort to ensure that all financial aspects are well organised. Luckily my wife and I had both paid into our pension schemes. It was very important to me that I left my wife in a good financial state; I felt that was the very least I could do for her.

After we signed the paperwork we discussed the financial planning, the implications the disease would have on my career, legal and insurance matters, and treatment logistics[20].

9 May 2022: Telling your friends and colleagues and final check-in with your career coach

BBC Headline: Prince Charles to deliver Queen's speech for the first time

By the time my wife and I returned from our hospital visit where we had been told about the brain tumour, I had made the decision to be open and honest with people. At the time, I was, obviously, in complete shock – this was the first time I was confronted with my own mortality. Nevertheless, I felt determined that this illness should not determine the rest of my life. One way to achieve this was to talk to friends and close colleagues. Over the next couple of weeks, I had many conversations with friends about my tumour. Their support was of great help to me.

The date 9 May 2022 will be a tough day. I had booked a series of video calls to inform my colleagues about my brain tumour. Some colleagues I wanted to inform simply because I could not support the project we were working on. Some colleagues I considered being my friends, so they should also know.

My first call started at 9:00 am, and my last call was supposed to end at 20:00 pm. Most calls were scheduled for 1 h. When I finally disconnected the last call, I felt an overwhelming feeling of being blessed. I had spoken about my tumour for most of the day. I received so much solid advice. The distinction between

---

[20] I refer the reader to Coping with cancer | Cancer Research UK for additional details.

colleagues and friends was blurred. I realised that different people could offer me different types of support.

I had my final meeting with my career coach. Career coaching was offered to all corporate employees to help them advance their careers. My coach and I had our first meeting in November, and we spoke at regular intervals during the intervening 6 months.

During our first session, my coach asked me the following questions:

Describe a few experiences that are magical, whatever magical means to you, and explain why they were magical.
Describe examples of what makes you feel annoyed/frustrated and/or angry and why.

What makes you happy and why?

I remember my attempt to answer these questions and how my coach created a list of my values. This will be used to identify a series of professional development goals consistent with my personal values.

Here are the values that my coach listed based on my answers, in decreasing order of importance:

1. Development and Growth
2. Quality of Life
3. Responsibility
4. Communication
5. Nature[21]
6. Reliability
7. Justice
8. Fairness
9. Respect
10. Integrity
11. Understanding
12. Control
13. Transparency

---

[21] The concept of nature to me means beauty, tranquillity, peace, and stillness.

50

I categorised these 13 values as follows:

1) *Development and Growth*, Responsibility, and Control
2) *Quality of Life*, Nature[22], Life
3) *Communication*, Reliability, Understanding, Transparency
4) *Fairness*, Justice, Respect, Integrity

In italics, I have indicated the term that I think somehow summarises the essence of the other words listed in each of the four categories.

Values 1 and 3 are operational values. Those values that must be successful in a corporate setting. Values 2 and 4 are much more personal[23].

In our last meeting, my coach and I reviewed the professional and personal journey had experienced during the previous 6 months. What I had learned about myself, what I will take forward, and what I will do more of. Typical exit questions. Once we worked our way down the questions, I paused and started asking about my personal values and asked her if anything distinguished me from my peers.

This puzzled her, and she asked me if I wanted to tell her something. I had not intended to share the news about my tumour, but her questions prompted me to share my health issues with her.

After a short pause, I asked her if there was anything that defined my colleagues as a group. Was there something that distinguished us from people who worked in, for example, finance, energy, or retail? I knew she was working on several coaching programmes that were offered to various companies operating in different industries. My coach reflected for a couple seconds and then replied that two things stood out. In my coach's opinion, my peers tended to be kind and caring and highly knowledgeable in their field of expertise.

My impression of the company four years ago was very different. I visualised the company as an island in the middle of the ocean, surrounded by sharks. On the island was the board of directors. The sharks represented senior management

---

[22] Now I am about to finish this book I have become attached to Nature a lot more since I wrote the first draft. Nature for now feels like it encapsulates the meaning of life...

23 Ralph Keeney, in his book "Value Focussed Thinking" refers to values 1 and 3 as "means to an end" – objectives that feed into the strategic objectives represented by values 2 and 4. To create a sustainable, enduring professional relationship between myself and my employer, values 2 and 4 must be satisfied.

desperate to engage with the board while keeping lesser mortals away from the island. Although I still believe that there is some truth in this mental image, my perspective over the last year has shifted closer to that of my coach.

I like to believe that all humans are decent – good at heart. I subscribe to Bergman's view[24] that even though horrendous crimes have been committed, humans have an intrinsic desire to make a positive contribution to the world. Sometimes stupid politics get in the way…

10 May 2022: Telling my brother and visiting Tesco in Sudbury

BBC Headline: Ukraine War: Putin gives few clues in Victory Day speech

51 days after my "suspected seizure" and 13 days after a CT scan showed a brain tumour, I spoke to my brother. On Friday last week, after my call with my sister-in-law, my brother dropped me a short message. I sent him a short reply, 'Not to worry about me.' I knew that this was not sufficient to calm his nerves. Last night, I mailed him a copy of the letter I wrote to my mother-in-law. I hoped that this letter would reassure both my brother and my sister-in-law that my wife and I had a grip on the situation.

Realising that we were about to start a very difficult conversation, I started by asking him how he felt. My brother spoke for the first 10–15 minutes. The information he provided allowed me to reassure him, and I answered his specific questions. My brother and I laid down some ground rules for future conversations: 1) We did not want the future conversation to be completely dominated by my illness, 2) We should be very clear to each other what type of support is needed and when, and 3) We should keep in touch.

We spoke for just over an hour. My brother told me how he had already started to prioritise non-work activities (dog training) and about his plans to buy a motorhome (well…there is a surprise[25]). I am sure that my illness has accelerated his decision making!

Ever since a tumour was identified on a CT scan of my brain, I have been hyper-sensitive to what really matters to me – what values are most important to me. It felt like being in an optician's chair having flicked a lens that suddenly transformed a fuzzy image into an incredibly sharp picture.

---

[24] Bregman, 2019

[25] My Grandfather and Dad have both owned motorhomes for the past 50 years.

I entered the Tesco store, hyper-aware of this new focus. I saw Tesco employees restocking shelves and pushing trolleys around, collecting items on their clients' shopping lists. I was wondering what their value functions looked like and whether they ever had given their objectives any serious thought. To me, it seemed like they were mindless robots moving through the store.

I was also very conscious of my wife's objectives. She just wanted to push her trolley through the shop, collect all her family's needs in the trolley, and leave the store with as little hassle as possible. She did not need my help with this task. So, I left her to it. I coaxed our son from his Mum and the trolley so that we could have our own conversation.

We ended up looking at four types of juice. I asked him which one he preferred. He was not interested in any juice, although I know that Tropical Juice is his favourite. I did care. As this could well be one of the last weeks that my brain has been working properly. I chose a bottle of orange juice "with bits"[26].

I took the bottle back to our trolley. My wife was in the aisle of breakfast cereals. I noticed that the brand I normally use was on offer and grabbed two bags. My wife gave me a disapproving look. I explained the discount, and she dropped the muesli into the trolley.

Most of us go through life in an almost dream-like state, our thoughts are mostly inward focused, and little of what we perceive has any relationship with objective reality.

The fact that Tesco is a very busy store despite having cheaper supermarket shops nearby implies that people are not solely focussed on saving money. This flaw in traditional economic theory was mentioned many decades ago. Economists talk about utility, of which money is one component. Utility, however, is still a one-dimensional metric (see chapter *Willingness to Pay*).

In the early 1990s, Ralph Keeney developed a practical framework that allowed the creation of a personal value system. These values are often conflicting, and the resulting trade-offs tend to complicate decision-making.

...Once we returned home, I found four unopened bags of muesli in the cupboard.

---

[26] Opposed to smooth juice without "bits".

11 May 2022: Coming to grips with hospital culture

BBC Headline: Deborah James: All I want are more life, says Big C presenter

When I was diagnosed with a brain tumour, I virtually had no experience with hospitals. I feel very ignorant about hospitals despite having been employed in the pharmaceutical industry for nine years. I started my professional career[27] in the early 2000s at H Lundbeck A/S, moved to Novo Nordisk, and after a break lasting just over a decade whilst being employed in the energy section, I returned to the pharmaceutical industry six years ago. The way hospitals are run, the way they are inward-looking, and their internal decision-making processes are completely alien to me.

The first major difference I discovered is that hospitals collect internal data for survival analysis. This is very different from the way pharmaceutical companies operate. Pharmaceutical companies realise that they cannot obtain access to patient data, so they rely on published data.

The fact that hospitals are inward looking should not come as a surprise. The entire hospital system is designed to help patients. Consequently, their view of the world is focussed on the care that the hospital provides to their patients. Data collected by a hospital focus on patients under their care. They have small datasets, so the issue of "small numbers" is very significant. Patterns in the data might be without meaning and totally spurious. The perceived "signal" might nevertheless trigger doctors to change the treatment regime.

Another key learning for me was that doctors do not speculate. Although decision making and the creation of judgements are fundamental tasks for doctors, they will simply not engage with patients if asked to create a judgement. Even though I have developed a rigorous method of expert. Doctors cannot share survival data because of patient confidentiality issues. My doctor reviewed the sources I used in my survival analysis but has not offered any assistance in adding academic papers that could strengthen the analyses. It came down to me, the patient, to judge my time of death and the Quality of Life I could expect. I received an estimate such as "you have 16 months to live" or an assessment "there is no visual sign of any cancerous growth". However, this leaves the question of whether the small cohort of patients that I was lumped into was

---

[27] Opposed to my academic career, which ended with a postdoctoral position in Germany.

appropriate. Did I truly belong to that cohort? Was I a representative sample of that population?

In the middle of May 2022, I wrote an email to the physician who found the tumour to express my gratitude to her. In her reply, she told me 'You are not a statistic!' I fundamentally disagreed with her at the time. However, now that I have experienced the way hospitals operate and reflected on this some more, I do understand where she is coming from.

Tetlock and Gardner, in their book *Superforecasting*, stated, 'It was the absence of doubt – and scientific rigour – that made medicine unscientific and caused it to stagnate for so long.' The authors dedicated a whole chapter to the historical treatments offered by so-called doctors and concluded that most of the treatments on offer reduced the health of the patients under their care. In his autobiography, *One Man's Medicine*, Archie Cochrane described the resistance of his fellow doctors when he tried to introduce scientific rigour by running early clinical trials in the 1950s and 1960s. In the same period, Cochrane was diagnosed with cancer, basal cell carcinoma. After Cochrane recovered from the operation, the treating physician told Cochrane that he had a terminal illness and will die shortly. Rather than challenging the doctor's judgement, Cochrane resigned to the diagnosis. This contradiction was stressed by Tetlock and Gardner: 'Why did a man who stressed the importance of not rushing to judgements accept the judgement of his fellow doctors that he had terminal cancer?'

12 May 2022: First version of an influence diagram

BBC Headline: Apple loses position as most valuable firm during tech sell-off

Archie the dog jumped on the bed. Our son followed Archie into our bedroom, and he was surprised to see me still in bed at 7 am. Our son asked why I was still in bed as my normal daily routine was getting up at 6:40. I explained that I needed some more sleep because I was taking medication for today's hospital appointment.

In preparation for the hospital appointment, I created an Excel file with a list of Givens, Uncertainties and Decisions. Some of the uncertainties listed are uncertainties to us, i.e., my wife and me, but are givens to the hospital, and some of the uncertainties are true uncertainties as neither the hospital staff nor we have the information to resolve the uncertainty. Figure 2.2 shows the first step in the construction of an influence diagram.

	A	B	C	D	E	F	G	H	I
1	Issues:								
2	Facts								
3		Brain tumour has been found							
4		Treatment plan has been selected							
5		Large uncertainties will persist for a long time (survival, QoL)							
6		Hospital is world class							
7	Uncertainties to us (but facts known to hospital)								
8		Treatment plan							
9			surgery - when, risks, time in hospital, expected side effects						
10			biopsy - how long do results take?						
11			post surgery: assessment of success of surgery, time before travel?						
12			radio therapy: start when? Duration						
13			chemo						
14			clinical trials						
15			full body MRI						
16		What are our decisions; what can we impact?							
17		Logistics of treatment (schedule, who is our contact person)							
18		Support for me and my wife							
19		Private insurance - can this be used to our advantage							
20		Advice on cognitive assessment (tracking decline)							
21	Uncertainties that persist (to both the hospital and us)								
22		Clinical outcome operation; headaches, seizures, tiredness, change of personality,..							
23		Prognosis - What do we know so far?							
24		What is the impact of having learned English as a second language							
25	Our decisions for now (what is in our control)								
26		How to use our private insurance money							
27		Change hospital							
28	Our decisions for later (what is in our control)								
29		Choose clinical trial							
30	To be discussed later								
31		Engage with AZ oncologist to stimulate collaboration with hospital							

Figure 2.2. Creation of an influence diagram, listing the givens,
uncertainties, and decisions.

I added a tab in the spreadsheet for each hospital visit to track how the decision situation evolved over time.

13 May 2022: Breaking the news to my parents

BBC Headline: Boris Johnson wants to cut up to 91,000 civil service jobs

A single guiding principle I set for myself: I did not want to tell my parents any lies. I would only allow myself to withhold some facts. The facts are very grim. Also, I needed to provide them with an accurate picture of the fact that I do have a brain tumour. I wanted to get the message to them before I became a patient. At that point, I became a patient, and I really needed to be able to focus on myself. The day I would turn into a patient was currently uncertain, but this uncertainty would be revealed the next day at 15:00 by the oncology department.

My Mum is 79 years old. Her mental state is fragile. A decline in her mental strength started 20–25 years ago but appears to have accelerated over the past couple of years. She just recovered from a hip replacement. My Dad turned 80 in March. Dad is not the easiest person. He started to suffer from terrible back pains in the 1980s when he was in his early thirties. Almost overnight, Dad became disabled and lost half his salary, and the culmination of these events triggered a long-lasting depression. Approximately 15 years ago, he was diagnosed with prostate cancer. Ironically, this event changed his life for the better. After a very stringent rehabilitation regime, Dad could have a normal life. However, the disabilities that affected him from his mid-thirties to his late sixties must have left him with some deep mental scars.

Dad was rushed to the hospital twice in the past year. His back pain had returned. The side effects of the large doses of opiates clouded his mind and judgement. In 2022, I travelled home several times to visit while navigating the ever-changing COVID-19 border crossing rules. It was very difficult for me to determine my parents in such a terrible state and realise that I would not be able to provide future support to them. My parents are still living in a large house on the outskirts of a small village in the south-eastern part of the Netherlands. A core objective of my Dad is to continue living his current life for as long as possible. I am terrified that my illness will throw a wrench at this plan.

At the time my tumour was discovered, my parents were travelling through southern France in their motorhome. We continued to communicate in our usual way. During their previous trips, Dad and I exchanged short WhatsApp messages once or twice a week. I understood that their vacation was not going to plan. Dad's pain increased to the point that they had to return home. The warm climate in southern France was no longer sufficient to ward off his pain. My sister-in-law told me that Mum and Dad would return home on Monday, May 9, 2022. On Monday, we exchanged a couple of messages. I told him that later this week, I would have a hospital appointment to receive some test results. I had never mentioned that I was getting medical tests done, and I am sure that my parents were aware of this.

Friday, May 13, 2022, was the day I told my parents.

Dad answered the phone. I asked him and Mum to sit down at the table. I dropped the bomb. I knew that after I told them 'I have a brain tumour,' their heads would be spinning and that no additional information would be absorbed.

I put down the phone and had an anxious wait for a couple of hours. I knew that both my brother and my sister-in-law were supporting my parents.

After 2 hours, I texted my sister-in-law. She called me on the speaker so my parents could hear me. I explained to my parents that I had known about the tumour for a couple of weeks and that I did not want them to hear this news while they were travelling through France. My sister-in-law prompted me, 'How do you feel?' As good as I could, I tried painting a positive picture of a bad situation. I told them about the quality of the medical team, the internal support network of colleagues, and the relevant knowledge that both my wife and I brought to the table.

After the phone call, I took Archie, the dog, for a 2-h walk. Once back, I called my parents. They were outside, fishing for small fish from their garden pond. I tried to gauge how they were coping with the bad news I had given them earlier that morning.

I was left unconvinced that they were honest.

14 May 2022: Chronic pain and the importance of routine

BBC Headline: Eurovision final 2022: Wolves, treadmills and high hopes for the UK

Early in the morning during my steroid-induced awakenings, I was thinking about my Dad. Dad was likely to be awake at the same time because of the same steroid side effects. Dad was in much pain. I read a BBC article stating that one in four people are living with chronic pain. BBC reported: 'Chronic pain, defined as pain that lasts longer than 3 months, can drastically change people's lives. It can be caused by a physical problem, such as a slipped disc, but can also occur with no clear cause, known as primary pain. It destroys careers, breaks up relationships, steals independence and denies people the futures they had imagined.

I felt fortunate. At this point in time, the brain tumour had not affected my Quality of Life, neither physically nor mentally.

20 days had passed since the consultant identified the tumour on the CT scan. These 20 days had been a maelstrom, a whirlwind of emotions. My wife and I had gone through the most intensive personal planning exercise in our lives.

Things that were fundamentally important to me had drastically changed. A seismic shock to my value system. It had taken me 20 days, but today I felt confident that we had left the storm behind us.

My line manager has been very clear to me that he did not expect anything workwise from me. However, I have had a very busy job for decades, and I am used to a consistent daily structure. In a post-COVID-19-lockdown world, I have become accustomed to booking online meetings. At this stage, I dropped all stressful calls and considered myself very fortunate that three or four stress-free meetings remained in my daily diary.

The continued routine was very important to me. I also started to think slightly longer term. I somehow needed to create opportunities to continue with my daily routine once I had sufficiently recovered from the operation to be functional.

15 May 2022: Talking to our daughter

At 6:30 in the evening, I was getting hungry and walked to my wife's office. I heard her talking to our daughter. Our daughter was clearly very upset. My wife spoke to her at a very slow pace trying to get all relevant information across to our daughter. I welled up. I walked to our living room and sat in silence for the next 20 min thinking about our daughter.

Our daughter's plans were to finish her first year at university, come home for a couple of days, work in a hotel on the Scottish west coast for a couple of months, and spend the final part of summer interrailing with one of her friends.

My wife and I are completely aligned in our view that our daughter needs to deal with this shock in her own way, and getting home immediately might simply not be the best idea. However, our daughter will need some help in making the right decisions. Our daughter needs support to get her life back on track after this shock. My wife is very well qualified to get her through these very turbulent days.

17 May 2022: Talking to our son

BBC Headline: Hundreds of fighters leave the Mariupol steelworks

Yesterday, after dinner, our son entered my office. I told him I was writing a biography and a diary. I showed him what I wrote on Sunday about his friends messing around and the fact that it had made me feel very happy.

I felt strongly that he should know the truth about what was happening to me. Our son told me that I would be fine after the operation. This was unlikely to be true. Our son did not really get his head around the fact that cancer can actually kill people. I told him that I was not worried about the operation but was concerned about the genetic makeup of the golf ball-sized tumour in my brain. Suddenly, the seriousness of the situation became clear to him. The tumour type would determine the time I had left with our son. At this very moment, I was unsure whether I had done the right thing – could I have delivered this message in any other, better, way?

Our son and I embraced each other in an emotional hug that lasted a long time. I told him that I loved him. That very day, I discovered that he had been looking at dirt bikes and pit bikes. I tried distracting him by looking at some online pictures of the bikes. Afterwards, he went to sit with his Mum and spent the next 10-15 minutes with my wife and Archie, the dog. At 22:30, more than an hour after his usual bedtime, he went to bed. I was unsure if I had done the right thing. I was fearful that our son might be at the beginning of a long sleepless night. Also, this felt like the first test of my newly found happiness.

I went downstairs to the living room and sat down in the same seat as I had sat on after I overheard a conversation between my wife and our daughter.

Today, I was awake at 3:30. For hours, I worried about our son. Our son is an early riser, and I went into his room just after 6:00. He was awake, looking at his phone.

Both of us were very emotional. We held our hands. I picked up a device that is used to increase the strength of your hands – a hand squeezer. Our son changed the toughness setting, and we squeezed the device in turns. We have continued our discussion on motor bikes.

We had breakfast. I have explained the distinction between tumour and cancer. I also told him that I was reasonably sure that one can undergo brain surgery only once. They cannot remove the tumour in its entirety and subsequent treatment is needed to kill any remaining cancerous cells.

After breakfast, our son, the dog, and I went for a short walk. Our first ever post-breakfast walk. We walked past the garden with one of the village friends. The couple was off-roading somewhere in southeast Europe. The dog entered their garden and dropped a poo in the middle of their garden. This was not the first time that that happened.

I felt that our son was coping very well with this very serious situation. My happiness had not changed in the last 24 h – I passed the first true test.

19 May 2022: Core Values

BBC Headline: Australia election: How climate is making Australia more unliveable

I spoke to the person who previously led our Biometrics and Information Sciences group. She interviewed me when I was a candidate to join the company. I was very keen to talk to her to get her thoughts on the challenges faced by decision sciences and what we could do as decision science professionals to enhance our impact. Her thoughts were very well structured. Everything she said made complete sense. I got some new ideas, some of which were debunked, and others were confirmed.

At the end of our conversation, I told her that she had been an inspiration to me. Before joining the pharmaceutical company, I had been working in the oil and gas industry for over a decade. The most important corporate core value in oil and gas energy is generally expressed as "safety first". The efforts made by oil and gas companies to reinforce these values in their onshore workforce always seemed somewhat dishonest to me. Every meeting began with a "safety moment". These safety briefs often involved short videos on a range of topics that had at best a tenuous link to safety.

On one occasion, the entire team was gathered in a meeting room. We were all asked to write down a safety pledge. After I made my statement, I never heard anything about it! Look, let's be clear. Every year, oil and gas employees perish on their jobs, so I understand the relevance of this core value. What upsets me is that the actions taken by staff employed in oil and gas are not consistent with the core value of "safety first".

During the preparation for my interview, I reread the company's core values (Figure 2.3):

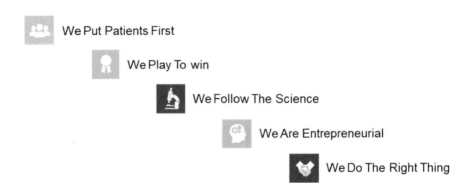

Figure 2.3. Core values of the pharmaceutical company.

At the time, I looked at them rather sceptically. I attempted to create an example for each of the five core values.

Once I joined the company and attended a couple of town halls, I realised that she was sincere about the company's most important core values: "We Put Patients First". After I mentioned to her that her sincerity was not left unnoticed, she shared with me that I would find the reasons behind her value system in a novel called *Sisters Pieced Together*. I ordered the novel, despite not having read a novel in many decades.

Over the past few weeks, my values have dramatically changed. Two core values resonate in particular: "We Put Patients First", and "We Follow The Science".

In recent years, I have applied for several jobs in the renewable energy sector. The main reason for not pursuing further opportunities in that space was that I would have to accept a significant cut in salary. However, because of the dramatic shift in my value system, I would not even consider returning to the energy sector. The company's core values are fully aligned with mine. In fact, very similar core values have been adopted throughout the pharmaceutical and biotech industries.

20 May 2022: Coping mechanisms

BBC Headline: Sue Gray planning to name No. 10 Covid rulebreakers

I recognise that people have different coping mechanisms. Each of these coping mechanisms is ultimately defined by a value system. In times of crisis, people revert to those beliefs that are intrinsically important to them, something that they have faith in.

One of my mum's aunts lit a massive candle for me, and I was given a little statue from Lourdes, which she also bought for me. One of my uncles led the prayers in church with my support. My parents and me brother have "hope" as a coping mechanism. "Hope" that I will somehow pull through, that the cancer will stop growing, and that I will stick around for another 3 decades. Other coping mechanisms include positive thinking, yoga, herbal medicines, and cancer support groups.

My coping mechanism is science and philosophy. I believe that through the pursuit of science and philosophy, we can not only find a cure for cancer but also solve many of the threats that we as humans are facing today[28]. None of the other coping mechanisms were ever a serious contender to me. As I have already stated, I believe that a coping mechanism is probably the closest one can get to a personal value system. It might even be that they are the same…

I am respectful of peoples coping mechanisms, and I would like to end with a quote from Volkan and Zintl[29]: 'Our griefs are as personal as our fingerprints.'

21 May 2022: Letter to my children

The day that Elon Musk spent 44 billion dollars on Twitter, my doctor told me that I had a brain tumour.

My wife was in the room when the doctor told us the news. My wife has a Ph.D. in pharmacology with a specific focus on neuroscience, and her father died of a brain tumour. So, if anything, she is much more knowledgeable than I am on brain tumours. There was no need to inform her – she knew the seriousness of the situation.

We told our son together, while my wife looked after sharing the devastating news with our daughter, who was away at university. Later, I decided that I also wanted to write a letter to the children, just in case surgery[30] didn't go to plan…

---

[28] Actions to combat climate change, the spread of misinformation, energy transition, the concentration of wealth, failing democracies, population growth, and the ethics of AI are all long overdue.

[29] Volkan and Zintl, 2015.

[30] A year later, this operation was followed by a second operation.

The hardest thing I have done in my entire life is writing a letter to my children. Realising that I had only a year, maybe a couple of years, left before my death. I was fully aware of the importance of that letter and this final letter to my children. I had to stop several times whilst writing the letter as I became overwhelmed with emotions. Saying farewell to your children is not easy...

What made the writing of the letter even harder was the fact that I felt a strong sense of guilt, feeling that I had not been completely honest – I felt I had withheld some crucial information about my life expectancy from them. I am not sure whether my children will ever forgive me for that.

Family is what really matters. My wife and children are by far the most important to me.

24 May 2022: Impact of cancer on my personal objective network

BBC Headline: Professor Brian Cox: Maybe humans are Martians

I have adapted Ralph Keeney's objective network to reflect my personal value system (see chapter *Values*). My life has been a rollercoaster during the past few months. Some values and objectives that were very important to me before I was diagnosed with cancer have lost their importance and are worthless to me now. Other values have become much more important to me. I have reprioritised my strategic objectives and added one objective. The one objective I have added is really important to me at this point – cancer should not affect the way I live my life. I am determined to ensure that my illness will have no impact on my family for as long as possible. The value of "Minimising the impact of cancer on family life" is the most important to me. "To enhance the life of family and friends" has become my second most important strategic objective. "To enjoy life" and "To be intellectually fulfilled" dropped to 3rd and 4th, respectively (see Figure 2.4). Therefore, although the main strategic objective "Happiness" has not changed, the objectives for achieving this have changed.

For some time, I questioned whether I had been too focussed on progressing my career, which was an attempt to fulfil my objective of "Maximise financial wellbeing". I do realise that there is a trade-off here. I chose to pursue a career that offered a higher salary and more opportunities for advancement. I have sacrificed time that I could have spent with my family and friends. I could have made a different choice. Taking a job that paid less, offered flexible hours, and left evenings free. No single choice is right or wrong. The choices made reflect personal preferences (Figure 2.5).

Pre-cancer diagnosis Strategic objectives: Maximise Happiness	Post-cancer diagnosis Strategic objectives: Maximise Happiness
To enjoy life To be intellectually fulfilled To enhance the life of family and friends	Minimise impact of cancer on family life To enhance the life of family and friends To enjoy life To be intellectually fulfilled

Figure 2.4. Strategic objective before and after cancer diagnosis

This reprioritization of objectives has resulted in a revision of my personal objective network. The objective network that I had until my brain tumour was identified in May 2022 is shown in Figure 2.5. The network features some objectives that were identified in the work I did with my career coach and several objectives that were identified by Ralph Keeney. This network reflects the objectives of an individual pursuing a strategy of establishing and maintaining a corporate network to gain access to promising projects. I have added personal core values pertaining to "fairness", "communication" and "We Put Patients First".

The objective "To maximise personal satisfaction" needs some explanations; I perceive it to be different from the strategic objective "Happiness". The objective "To maximise personal satisfaction" refers to one of my core beliefs that I cannot help other people with their "Happiness" if I am unhappy myself. It is only when that value has been satisfied that I can truly engage with the objective "To pursue worthwhile activities & collaborations".

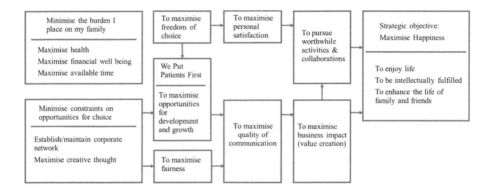

Figure 2.5. My personal objective network before cancer.

The diagnosis of a brain tumour caused a seismic shock to my value system. At this very moment, "health" and "time" are synonymous. I have a visual image of my brain as a bomb that is likely to explode in six to twelve months. Time has become my most precious resource. The problem with survival time is that it is uncertain. I might die in 2 months, or I might still be alive five years from now.

There are numerous differences between the two strategic objective networks (Figure 2.5 and Figure 2.6). Although the starting point (the two boxes on the left upper part of the diagram) and the strategic objectives (the box on the far right) have been only marginally affected, the remaining objectives have dramatically changed. Objectives that were highly relevant only a couple of months ago have been removed from the network while new objectives have been identified. One mechanism to achieve the objective of "minimising the impact of cancer on family life" is to ensure that I remain busy. Therefore, I set myself a writing challenge. The writing challenge will hopefully prevent me from getting bored – English winters are very long.

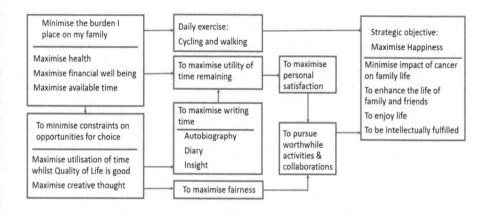

Figure 2.6. My personal objective network immediately after cancer diagnosis.

28 May 2022: Doing too much...

BBC Headline: Bristol Mayor Flies Nine Hours for TED Climate Conference

At 10:30 a.m., an Irish village friend came over to take down a branch in our back garden. A conifer branch broke away at a height of about 6 m, and given my current condition, I did not want to climb up a ladder to cut it loose. My friend used a handsaw to cut down the branch. Once the branch was on the ground, he used my chainsaw to chop the wood into logs that would fit into my woodburning stove. Together, we stacked the wood into the woodshed.

By the time we were done, it was 13:30, time for lunch. At that stage, I felt a slight unease in my stomach. I assumed that I had become nervous at a subconscious level because my surgery was planned in 2 days' time. Over the next hour or so, the pain in my stomach became more intense. Suddenly, I emptied my stomach. I ran to the bathroom and made a mess in the hallway and the bathroom. I realised that this must have been a shock to my family. Then I realised that these stomach pains were not nerves. I had simply done too much. I had a very busy morning. Moving the wood, trimming grass, and taking a cold shower (we ran out of hot water) were the likely causes of my stomach pain.

I withdrew to the bedroom. I lay in bed for several hours. I tried to recover by drinking water and eating some nuts and raisins.

29 May 2022: 1 day before the operation

BBC Headline: Why can't the US stop soaring oil and gas prices?

As usual, I woke up early in the morning. I was conscious that I needed to recover from yesterday's episode. I got up to get some orange juice and nuts. At 8:00 am, I prepared some fruit and yogurt. Followed by two slices of bread with jam and honey.

I continued with Bart van Loo's book on Napoleon. I spend several hours reading. I read about Austerlitz, and how he moved his troops east towards Russia.

After lunch, I marinated the meat for a BBQ. I figured I could also do with some carbohydrates because I was not supposed to eat anything after midnight and was not allowed a drink after 6:00 am Monday because of the operation. The whole situation reminded me of the situation of inmates on death row in the US when they can choose their final meal. My choice: meat, salad, and pasta.

I am not worried about the operation tomorrow. It does feel a bit unreal. Tomorrow, a surgeon will be poking in my skull, pushing a bit of my brain tissue aside to cut away a golf ball-sized tumour. I really hope the surgeon has a steady hand.

I have not revised my estimates of long-term survival. I still believe that my P10, P50, and P90 estimates are accurate.

The next day, I reported to the hospital reception at 7:00 am.

3 June 2022: New scars

BBC Headline: Bart Willigers survived a brain tumour operation[31]

First whole day at home. I sat out in the sun for most of the day. I made my way through a decent part of my book narrating about Napoleon. I also had lunch and supper outside.

In the evening, I had a shower and noticed my new scar.

9 June 2022: Elicitation post biopsy results

BBC Headline: Europe's "largest ever" land dinosaur found on the Isle of Wight

On Thursday, June 9, 2022, I was diagnosed with glioblastoma. I was given 16 months to live. Glioblastomas are grade 4 brain tumours. Glioblastomas are

---

[31] ...I did not record what the BBC headline was...

fast growing and diffuse. Glioblastomas have thread-like tendrils that extend into other parts of the brain. Tumours may return and are difficult to treat. Glioblastomas are a type of glioma that is a brain tumour that grows from a glial cell. A glial cell is a type of brain cell that supports and protects nerve cells (neurons) in the brain by providing them with oxygen and nutrients.

The six years I had given myself were reduced to just 16 months by this diagnosis. The rationale behind these 16 months is that my brain tumour is very aggressive and difficult to treat.

I have a hunch that the doctors played a double act – good cop, bad cop – with me. The doctor who told me that I had 16 months left to live, I have never seen again after she poured a bucket of ice water over me. The doctor who ended up treating me left me with a much more comfortable feeling. He talked about "stunning the cancer" and "we will get you through the next 6 months."

Once I had my diagnosis, I knew what to look for online. One of my colleagues, who is a statistician, looked up 10 studies[32] that involved patients who suffered from a glioblastoma. After digitising the survival curves[33], I created two curves: one for Progression Free Survival and one for Overall Survival (Figure 2.7)[34]. Progression Free Survival is defined as the time it takes before the tumour starts to grow again. Overall Survival is time to death. A very dire outlook indeed…

---

[32] Roa et al. (2004, 2015), Hegi et al. (2005), Stupp et al. (2005, 2015), Minniti et al. (2009), Stupp et al. (2009), Malmström et al. (2012), Perry et al. (2017), Balana et al. (2020), Zur et al. (2020), and Zhang et al. (2020).

[33] https://automeris.io/WebPlotDigitizer/

[34] The curves are shown.

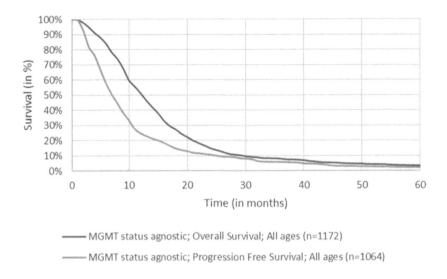

— MGMT status agnostic; Overall Survival; All ages (n=1172)
— MGMT status agnostic; Progression Free Survival; All ages (n=1064)

Figure 2.7. Overall survival versus Progression Free Survival.

Already after the first month post diagnosis, patients start to suffer. The Progression Free Survival curve drops at a constant rate for the first 11 months. At that point, 30% are progression-free. At this point, the survival curve becomes less steep and there is a long flat tail: the happy few that have survived the onslaught.

The Overall Survival curve is smooth. The rate of death increased over the first 6 months, remained constant for about a year, and slowly declined after a year and a half. After a year and a half, the Overall Survival rate is about 30%, further declining to 10% after thirty months.

4 July 2022: First day of my treatment

BBC Headline: Breast cancer drug trial: Woman given months to live told she is cancer free

This will be the first day of my treatment. Today, I will start with radiation therapy, and tomorrow, I will start chemotherapy. Clearly, there is uncertainty about how my body will react to a combined exposure to radiation therapy and chemotherapy. I might feel very tired and me body might feel terrible, or I might be absolutely fine, suffering from no side effects at all.

I found a headline that read: 'Breast cancer drug trial; Woman given months to live told she is cancer free.' The article recites a story about a woman who has been given months to live and is suddenly declared cancer free. This story is clearly completely anecdotal. Realistically, there is only a small probability that there will be a news story like this in a couple of months regarding my recovery.

08 July 2022: Influence diagram

BBC Headline: Boris Johnson: Tories vie for leadership as race to replace PM begins

In the second week of June 2022, I updated my influence diagram (Figure 2.8). The three types of issues are depicted as follows: givens are represented by diamonds, uncertainties are shown as rectangles with rounded corners, and decisions appear as rectangles with square corners[35]. The diagram shows three "givens": I have been diagnosed with a "Glioblastoma grade 4", "Tumour has been removed", "No reduction in QoL in the first chemo cycle". "Glioblastoma grade 4" was an uncertainty. However, biopsy analysis determined that the tumour was indeed a glioblastoma grade 4, thereby transforming that uncertainty into a given. The removal of the tumour is an example of a decision that was made by the clinical team.

The diagram depicts seven uncertainties. The one uncertainty that has input, but no output is "Happiness". Happiness is uncertain because it is unknown how the disease will progress, "Disease progression". The uncertainty "Disease progression" is directly influenced by three uncertainties: "MRI scan" and "Headaches, seizures, tiredness, memory loss, change of personality" and "Body's reaction to increased dose".

The two remaining uncertainties, "Other available treatments" and "Outcome second brain operation", are categorised as "for later" and thus are without connections because they do not yet influence the decision analysis.

The uncertainty "Happiness" is connected to a single decision: "Prioritisation of tasks", which would drive other choices I might need to make. The tasks I identified are shown in the section *September 2022 to December 2022: Attempts to draw a decision tree*. I also listed four decisions for later: "Decide on a second brain operation", "Retrieving information on clinical trials", "Retrieve driving

---

[35] I used the basic functionality of PowerPoint to draw this influence diagram but drawing them manually would often suffice.

license" and "Preparations for death". As these four decisions were not part of the current focus, they were kept unconnected by arrows, i.e., they are not an integral part of the immediate decision.

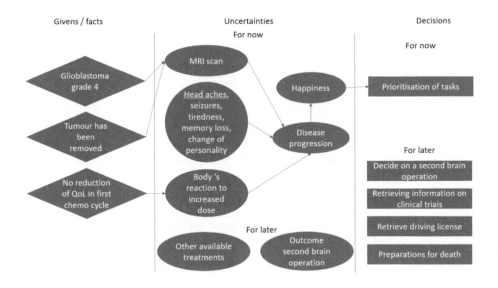

Figure 2.8. Influence diagram listing the given, uncertainties and decisions.

14 July 2022: Our son's birthday

BBC Headline: Jurassic Coast heatwave rockfall warning

Our son's birthday! I woke up early this morning to determine whether he was already awake. And he was – so I congratulated him! I did some work in the morning. These days "work" is writing my blog and sorting out slides. The four of us went to Cambridge in the afternoon. We first went to the hospital for the usual radiation therapy session, and then we went to a sushi restaurant for a bite to eat. On the way back, we split. My wife and I went to buy oil for our son's new pit bike, which was due to arrive this week, and the children went to buy birthday cake!

Spending time with my family has become very valuable to me because I know that I do not have much time left. I do feel a strong sense of guilt towards my children – guilt that I have taken them for granted for too long…

15 July 2022: The radiation routine

BBC Headline: Heatwave: Nantwich ice cream firm Snugburys doubles production

It is Friday again – another week over. It never stops astonishing me how quickly one gets used to a new routine. Especially when a routine is completely bizarre, such as visiting the hospital every weekday for radiation therapy.

I received chemotherapy before being taken to the hospital. Two little tablets of poison. One 140 mg and a second one 5 mg. Today, I was driven to the hospital by our daughter. I was dropped off at the main reception and continued my way to the oncology department. During the walk through the hospital, I noticed "thank you"-notes pinned up on the walls. These notes were illustrated using the familiar NHS-rainbow. A rainbow requires a combination of sunlight and rain. I was wondering whether this combination was the inspiration behind the NHS rainbow. The sun might be shining, but you still get soaking wet! I walked past a large waiting area with many seats. Most of them were empty. This image of all these seats reminded me of a factoid that I had read some time ago. Apparently, over 95% of oncology patients believe that their chance of survival is better than that of their fellow patients. I believe this is the case. This must be a prime example of *Survivorship bias*. In fact, in Rolf Dobelli's book *The Art of Thinking Clearly,* Survivorship bias is featured in the first chapter. Rolf ends the chapter with the following: 'Survivorship bias means that people systematically overestimate their chances of success. Guard against it by frequently visiting the graves of once-promising projects, investments, and careers. It is a sad walk, but one that should clear your mind.

Once I made my way past all these empty seats, I could see the sign that reads "radiation therapy reception". I walked up to the reception and said my name. I got into the habit of spelling it out because I am pretty confident that I am the sole patient called "Willigers" and I am all too familiar with Brits misspelling my surname – the most common error is to put an "n" between the "i" and the "g". Invariably, I am directed to either waiting room 7 or 8. I take a seat in a small waiting area with about ten chairs.

A nurse comes in and asks me at what time I have taken my pills. The thought that I simply might have forgotten to take my medication never seems to occur to the nurses. Approximately 5 minutes after the "medication reminder" I am picked up by a nurse who leads me to the room in which the radiation therapy takes place. The central feature in the room is a large machine that delivers the x-rays in a narrowly focussed beam precisely where the cancerous cells are located. In front of the machine is a large moveable bed. On this bed, I lay down and have my mask fitted. The mask fits really tightly. I close my eyes before the mask is pinned down. I hear the nurses communicating with each other: 'We have gone "soup" 1.4, "south" 3.' Once my head is secured in place, the nurses leave the room. I spend the next 10 minutes alone with the buzzing radiation machine. The procedure starts by moving the bed in the correct position. Once the position is fixed, I can hear a weird humming sound, which seems to come from all directions. I am at the receiving end of the x-rays. Even if I concentrate really hard, I cannot hear any popping noises of exploding cancer cells.

Once the humming sound stops and I hear a friendly voice saying, 'all done.' I get off the bed slowly. I am always expecting to faint when I get up. Once I am off the bed, I gather my personal belongings while conversing with the nurses. The questions they ask me; 'What are your plans for the weekend?', are all open questions, so one cannot answer them with a single word "Yes" or "No" answer. Trying to make conversation with cancer patients. I feel sorry for these nurses. I honestly think that they have made a bad choice in life. No one should be a nurse helping cancer patients. Brain cancer, like many other cancer types, has a very poor prognosis, and the chance of survival is very low. It is hard to imagine that of all patients, the nurses help very few patients who will still be around in two years...

I walk back through the corridors to find our daughter. I see her sitting in the entrance hall of the hospital. She is still wearing a face mask. I did not want to discuss my chances of surviving this ordeal.

21 July 2022: One of my closest friends has prostate cancer

BBC Headline: Whisky makers are turning their backs on peat

Last week, I received a call from one of my closest friends. After the customary small talk, my friend told me that he had been diagnosed with prostate cancer. The day we spoke, it was day four after my friend heard his diagnosis.

At the end of this initial phone call, I told him that we should make a follow-up call. That call took place today. I told my friend that I had been reading Keeney's Value-Focused Thinking. I looked up Keeney's personal fundamental value system and noticed that his fundamental value is "maximise happiness".

Clearly, prostate cancer is very different from a brain tumour; therefore, there are many more options available to patients who have been diagnosed with prostate cancer. Prostrate is also a much better understood disease. Depending on the findings of the biopsy, one can choose whether, for example, hormone treatment is the best choice.

We spoke for a full hour and promised each other that we would keep in contact.

22 July 2022: An easy decision to go back to work

BBC Headline: Ukraine and Russia sign 'beacon of hope' food crisis deal

I spoke to my line manager and told him that I wanted to return to work. The prime reason for my desire to return to work was that by working again, I would cause minimal disruption to my wife and my two children. Also, I felt that although the odds were stacked against me, I might, just might, be lucky enough to survive for another couple of years, and sitting at home doing nothing during the upcoming winter would drive me insane.

This was one of the easiest decisions I ever made!

26 July 2022: Laura Nuttall and her bucket list challenge

BBC Headline: Laura Nuttall presents the weather in cancer bucket list challenge

This morning, I was fiddling with my hair and suddenly noticed that I had a handful of hair in my hand. I looked at myself in the mirror and noticed a bald patch on the left side of my skull.

A real tragedy: 'A student who was given 12 months to live after being diagnosed with brain cancer has achieved another of her lifelong ambitions: to present the BBC weather forecast.

Laura Nuttall, from Barrowford, Lancashire, was diagnosed with glioblastoma multiforme after a routine eye test in 2018. She was later found to have eight tumours.

Ever since, 22-year-old Laura has been working her way through her bucket list and has met Michelle Obama, commanded a Royal Navy ship, and taken Peter Kay to a pub for drinks.

She recently graduated from the University of Manchester with a political science, philosophy, and economics degree.

Now she's visited the BBC's studios in Salford and, with a little help from weather presenter Owain Wyn Evans, presented her first forecast.'[36]

Being a 22-year-old – an adult for just four years – Laura has simply not lived long enough to realise all life's opportunities beyond the bucket list items she selected. Me on the other hand, being in my 50s, have had 3 decades to realise all my youthful dreams. I have lived as an adult.

3 August 2022: My birthday

BBC Headline: Driest July in England since 1935 – Met Office

My birthday – I am 52 years old today!

We ate birthday cake for lunch. I also got a present. We will see Professor Brian Cox that very same day. I was somewhat surprised by my emotional reaction – I felt like I was welling up. I finished my birthday cake. At 13:00, we set off for London. The plan was to have a steak before going to the theatre to watch Brian's show. Brian did his usual thing, quoting very large numbers – the age of the universe 13.8 billion years, the 3 trillion stars in the observable universe. He spoke about black holes and worm holes. He ended with a reference to Richard Feynman, a famous American physicist. Brian told his audience that science is the way forward; scientific thought can help mankind solve the biggest problems and navigate the various crises that are currently dominating the news headlines.

I snoozed in the car on the way back. My brain was spinning, not about the technical content of Brian's talk but more so about his final statement about the importance of science. I subscribe to the view that if we want to have a place to live 1000 years from now, we better get our act together sooner rather than later.

It crossed my mind that it would be interesting to determine the chance that I will reach my next birthday, but then I figured that that assessment is pointless and frankly too depressing.

9 August 2022: Life moves on

BBC Headline: Climate change: Alps glaciers melting faster as heatwaves hit

A friend from the village drove me to the hospital this morning. My friend was very apologetics when I stepped into his car. Over the next 10 min or so, the

---

[36] Laura died on the 22nd of May 2023. https://www.bbc.co.uk/news/uk-england-lancashire-65460230

reason for his anxiety gradually dawned on me. He was convinced that I had an 8:00 am appointment. Unknown to him, my appointment was an hour later at 9:00 am. So, I knew that although we left a little late, we could still be there in time, while my friend was convinced that I would arrive an hour late! I could have made him suffer all the way to Cambridge, but, being a nice person, I told him about the mix-up.

On the way back, we stopped at our usual café for breakfast and cappuccinos. After our break, we drove back to our village, and when we left the car park, I realised that my friend and I had just had a normal conversation – the topic of cancer was not discussed once!

11 August 2022: The law of small numbers

BBC Headline: Every day it doesn't rain, the pressure mounts

My wife and I met with my consultant. It appears that we are still waiting for genetic screening data. I was told that the fact that we do not have a complete genetic dataset has no impact on the next steps of my treatment. We have discussed the next phase of my treatment. I will be subjected to adjuvant chemotherapy. The adjuvant treatment, or secondary treatment, consists of six-monthly cycles in which the patient takes chemotherapy tablets for the first five days and the remainder of the month is dedicated to recovery.

In his book *Thinking, Fast and Slow,* Kahneman describes variations in the incidence rates of kidney cancer across US counties. Incidence rates are most variable in rural and sparsely populated Republican states in the Midwest, South, and West. It is easy to infer that the higher incidence rate is related to the rural lifestyle. No access to good medical care, a high-fat diet, excessive alcohol consumption, and excessive tobacco smoking. The incidence rates are not high in each state; in some states, rates are actually low. Although the logical inference that lifestyle choices result in a high incidence rate is simply false. System 1 provides a rational explanation for the facts and a solution that may sound logical, but it is in fact wrong. This is an example of the *law of small numbers*.

I wonder how many brain tumour patients the hospital has in total and is the hospital truly able to harness itself against the *law of small numbers*?

12 August 2022: A more sustainable objective network

BBC Headline: Sainsbury's and Tesco stop selling disposable barbecues

Last day of radiation treatment! After the treatment, my driver, a village friend, and I went to Cambridge to celebrate with sushi and beer.

At the end of July, I gradually started to realise that the value system I had created was not suitable for future living (Figure 2.6). I cannot live like this – it is simply too strenuous, too difficult.

I constructed an updated objective network, as shown in Figure 2.9. This figure is a hybrid of the two previous objective networks shown in Figures 2.5 and 2.6.

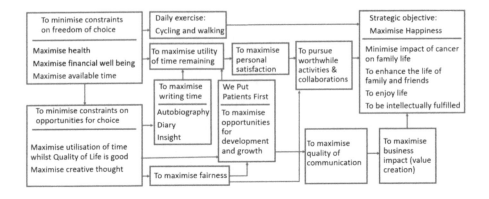

Figure 2.9. My personal objective network after dealing with the shock of cancer diagnosis.

Despite the odds, 7% of patients with my diagnosis are still alive after 5 years. I realised that I need to be prepared for this eventuality. Five years is a long time to nothing – way too long! The objective network I designed shows a balance between "writing time" and "We Put Patients First".

The moment I finished drawing this diagram (in mid-August 2022), I felt convinced that I had made the right decision to return to work. I need the daily routine that work provides and the mental challenges provided by both writing down my thoughts and executing decision analysis projects. After an absence of 3 months, I returned to my job at the beginning of September 2022. My job provides structure to my day and a reason to get up in the morning. I just must ensure that I don't spend too many hours working.

Overnight, I have become a prolific writer. I have so many ideas that I feel really passionate about, and I am not sure whether I have sufficient time left to finish my stories. I simply want to share my story with as many people as possible.

1 September 2022: First day back at work and I decided not to attend the Oslo conference

BBC Headline: Bill Turnbull obituary: Beloved BBC Breakfast host

Today is the first day that I am officially back at work. On the doctor's note, a box is ticked: "A phased return to work". It is up to me to decide how many hours per week I work. How many working days a week would be suitable to achieve the right balance between "working" and "writing"? Currently, I am inclined towards working 3 or 4 days a week. Also, I must suggest how often we revisit whatever we decide upon.

In the evening, I wrote an email informing the organising committee of the Decision Analysis/Decision Quality conference in Oslo that I wish to be relieved of my duties. This felt at the time like a hard decision to make. However, given that my doctor simply could not guarantee that I would have the stamina for a weeklong conference, the decision was straightforward – I simply had no choice. This was not a valid decision as I only had a single option available to me…

I had been looking forward to this event for months. I blocked out an entire week in my diary to accommodate the conference. I was surprisingly rational about my decision. I do recognise that I have been giving up so many things over the past months that not attending the conference is just one more additional thing. The conference will be over in a few weeks. I will have missed some happy memories, but this will not dramatically change my happiness in the long term.

14 September 2022: Having the courage to live

BBC Headline: Queen's coffin rests at palace ahead of lying-in-state

It has been 13 days since I wrote my previous entry in my diary. The reason for this break, the fact that I made no entry for nearly two weeks, is a change in my state of mind. During the two weeks I was on holiday, I finally managed to get beyond the shock of having been given 16 months to live. Dealing with this statistical reality is largely, or even entirely, beyond my control. I could not simply continue living as normal. I was simply unable to force myself to move on as if nothing had happened. Even as I write these words, I am fully aware that a cancer diagnosis is a life sentence. In my mind, there is a very clear distinction between before and after the CT scan. The image showing my brain tumour. The carefree state of the world experienced by me before the CT scan will never return. I do not expect there will be a single day in the future when I will not worry about the return of the tumour.

At some point last week, I actually don't remember when this thought first struck me, but I suddenly realised that it takes a lot of courage to enjoy life in the face of death. We all know that a fundamental consequence of life is death[37]. Death to me was something that happened to old people, and I am not old yet – I am still "relatively young" as one young doctor polity described my age.

The likelihood of dying at some stage in the next year of someone in his early fifties is just over half a percent. Personally, I consider this likelihood to be at least one order of magnitude too small to raise any reason for concern. After a brain tumour was identified, I was given a 93% chance of dying of a cancer at some stage over the next five years. Somehow, I needed to be prepared for the 7% likelihood that I would be around for another five years. I was fully aware that my mental state, my value system, over the summer was not sustainable in the long term. I needed to prepare a long-term plan for the future, no matter what the future had in store for me. Crucial to this plan was that it had the right balance of objectives: family and friends and intellectual stimulating project. I had a strong desire to live again.

What makes the situation incredible hard to comprehend is the complete lack of physical suffering – I don't feel any different from three, six, or even twelve months ago. Over the weekend, we visited a friend who was diagnosed with throat cancer. He cannot take in solid food. He was drinking liquids with a very specific viscosity – not too fluid and not too viscous – so he could swallow his food. Another friend of mine has been diagnosed with prostate cancer. I suspect that his prostate has been removed. I have not asked my friend the question, but if this operation was the same as that of my Dad, he would no longer be able to have an erection. My situation is very different. Although I have cancer as well, to this day, the treatment I have received has not affected my physical or mental abilities. This lack of physical and mental limitations makes me feel both guilty and very fortunate at the same time.

Yesterday, I had an MRI scan. The purpose of this scan I was told by my doctor was to be used as a "base line". I was not sure whether this was a euphemism, i.e., was the doctor expecting to see multiple cancer growths or was

---

[37] Although most of us are in denial of this reality.

the doctor sincere in getting a "base line"-image. I drafted a message for my doctor asking him what I should expect to see on the scanned image. I did not send the message. I deleted the message because I did not want to put my doctor in an awkward position. My doctor might not want to speculate without having a scan image on which to base his judgement. I did not sleep well the following night.

This morning, there was a planned power cut. My wife very kindly offered to drive me to the office, so I could meet up with some of my colleagues. I arranged four back-to-back meetings between 10:00 and 13:00. During my office visit, I ran into two colleagues and asked them whether they had any Decision Analysis projects for me. Both said yes! I also published an article on WorkPlace, the company's internal social media platform, in which I announced the launch of a web page dedicated to Decision Sciences. I had taken six years, but finally I was making some inroads. Although my illness might prevent me from finishing the work associated with these opportunities.

On the way back, the phone rang, and it was our neighbour. Due to the power cut, our gates did not open, and she had taken the delivery of a parcel. I walked into their house and noticed a fresh bunch of flowers on the kitchen table. These flowers were the parcel to which our neighbour referred. I took the flowers and handed them to my wife, as I was pretty sure that the bunch of flowers was not for me. She read the note, and to our surprise, the flowers were sent by my brother and his wife – a very thoughtful gesture.

28 September 2022: I am feeling great–despite the treatment

BBC Headline: Nord Stream leaks: Sabotage to blame, says EU

On Monday the 26th of September, I finished my first cycle of adjuvant chemotherapy. I consider myself very fortunate to have suffered no side effects apart from losing some hair, losing some sleep, and getting a bit constipated. I feel not different from the day I started taking chemo.

I hired an editor to help me write my autobiography. Yesterday afternoon, I searched for ghost-writers and approached several individuals. There is a whole world out there of people who offer their services for all writing styles. I selected my editor because I liked her profile and she is based in the United Kingdom. Therefore, I made the arrangement for her to be the ghost writer of my biography[38]. It is really important to me that the story of my life is being told in the best possible way. I feel the need to have a project to keep me going. I feel there is a need for me to stay busy over the winter. I am very aware that I might not survive this winter.

Tomorrow, it will be 6 months since I handed over my diving licence to the DVLA[39].

16 November 2022: A message to my friends

BBC Headline: Ros Atkins on… Is the 1.5C climate target still possible?

On 16 November 2022, I decided to play a morbid version of Michael McIntyre's "Send to All" from his Big Show. I have emailed all the people featured in my biography and told them about my current health condition:

Hi,

I have to tell you something, and I realise that this will come as a shock to you.

In the spring, I collapsed in the garden. I was rushed to the hospital, and the nurse told me I had a suspected stroke.

After further investigations, the doctors found a brain tumour. In July, the tumour was removed. In August, I was diagnosed and given 16 months to live.

I realise that this news will be a shock to you, but at the moment, I am doing well. I have had no more seizures; I have no pain, and I am not tired.

Bart

This short message triggered an avalanche of emails and phone calls. I was really surprised by the impact I made on other people – I am forever grateful.

---

[38] At this time, I focussed on writing my biography and my diary. Later in the autumn, it is decided to write this book.

[39] Driver and Vehicle Licensing Agency

September 2022 to December 2022: Attempts to draw a decision tree

BBC Headline: House prices see the biggest fall for two years, says Nationwide

During the autumn of 2022, I made several attempts at naming uncertainties and creating a list of discrete outcomes (Figure 2.10).

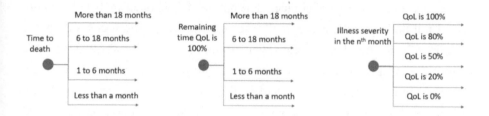

Figure 2.10. Three attempts at naming uncertainty and defining its outcomes.

I decided to go with the uncertainty shown on the right. The rationale behind this choice was that I wanted an uncertainty with a set of outcomes that would trigger different actions, and I felt that discrete scenarios "Quality of Life" would best accomplish this.

I did not experience any symptoms. I was however convinced that sooner or later these symptoms would have an impact. Hence, I also included a second uncertainty: the month in which I would experience the first symptoms of disease progression (Figure 2.11).

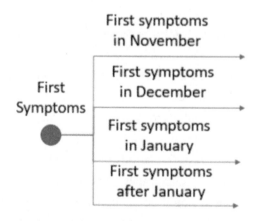

Figure 2.11. Uncertainty as to the first month in which I would be experiencing disease progression.

The timing of the first symptoms is a continuous uncertainty. The first symptom can occur at any moment. Therefore, I subdivided time into discrete, mutually exclusive scenarios. The final category "first symptoms after January" contains all scenarios in which the first symptoms were diagnosed in February or later. This includes a scenario where the first symptoms were diagnosed in March, for example.

Finally, I needed a set of choices. The options I developed are listed in Figure 2.12. I felt that I could engage in all five activities when life was good, that is, "Quality of Life" was 100%. I knew that ultimately my health would deteriorate. I anticipated that I would stop working and cycling first, but I would continue to socialise with my family, write, and walk. Once the disease progressed even further, I would stop writing and walking, but I would continue to socialise with my family. Finally, I would die.

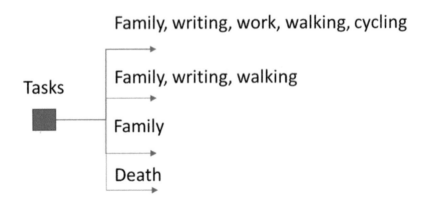

Figure 2.12. A list of choices available to me.

Figure 2.13 shows a decision tree with two uncertainties: the timing of the first symptoms and severity of these symptoms, and a single decision node: "tasks." Uncertainties are indicated by circles, and decisions are indicated by squares.

The decision node, "tasks", has also not been fully developed. I only developed the upper branch. Given that "QoL is 100%" or "Quality of Life is 100%", the optimal choice would be the upper branch: "Family, writing, work, walking and cycling". This branch is shown in bold. This bold branch indicates the optimal choice for a given outcome from the uncertainty resolved. In scenarios with lower QoL, different alternatives become optimal.

84

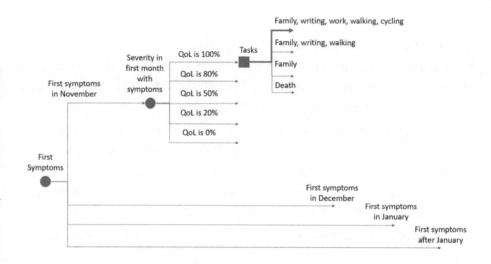

Figure 2.13. Example of an exploding decision tree that has been partly developed.

As illustrated in Figure 2.13, one of the problems with a decision tree is that it tends to grow exponentially in size. The decision tree shown above has not even been fully developed. As a rule of thumb, I would recommend that if the decision tree does not fit on a single A4, 21 x 29.7 cm, it is too big. In this case one should simplify the decision tree by removing some branching – clarity is the ultimate goal.

One aspect that is missing from this decision tree is how the severity develops after the first month has passed. The expectation is that the second month will be worse than the first month, ultimately ending in the inevitable outcome: "death".

Given all these issues I decided that this decision tree was not useable. The main concern I had with this decision tree was that regardless of my Quality of Life, it would not change the decisions I would make. I would like to continue with my current daily routine for as long as I can physically and mentally.

Finally, I also considered starting with the decision – Tasks. Followed by the uncertainties in order that they would be resolved. I did not pursue this option because, in my judgement this approach did not yield any helpful insight. I would still be doing what I am currently doing – "Family, writing, work, walking, cycling" – also this approach still does not allow for a reduction of the number of scenarios.

So, I scrapped this effort and started again!

Although I wasted some efforts, I did gain one important insight. I now knew that my preferences would not change. I would continue doing what I was already doing, regardless. Hence, there was no need for a decision node in the decision tree. I then drew a probability tree whose left-most input would be my estimate that an MRI scan on the 5th of December 2022 would indicate no new cancer growth, as shown in Figure 2.14.

For the uncertainty of *Overall Survival* I defined three point estimates – a P10, a P50, and a P90. In decision analysis, "P90" designates the true value that one believes has a 90% chance of being lower than the true value, "P10" designates the true value that one believes has a 90% chance of being higher than the true value, and "P50" designates an estimate that one is indifferent whether the true value is higher or lower. This tree was simple and would structure the output I was interested in – the length of my remaining life.

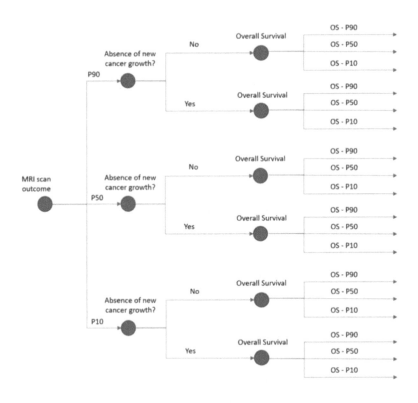

Figure 2.14. The probability tree is formulated for further analysis.

The only thing missing in this probability tree are the probabilities themselves. I planned to use expert elicitation to create a judgement of the uncertainty *on December 5, 2022, March 27, 2023, and June 26, 2023: Three revisions of chance of success.* I applied the methods described in the *Human Judgement* section to create a judgement on whether there were signs of cancer growth visible on the MRI scan images.

For the remaining two uncertainties, *MRI outcome* and *Overall Survival*, I consider the Upside and Downside cases as P90 and P10, respectively. In doing so, we can apply *Swanson's mean*. Following Swanson's mean, probability weighting is applied that assigns a 30% chance to both the P10 and P90 events and a 40% chance to the P50[40].

3 October 2022: Estimating the length of time to write a book

Saturday morning, the 3rd of October 2022, I took Archie for a walk. One of my favourite walks is a loop that takes you from the village where we live towards Stansfield, Suffolk. After I had given a biscuit to the dog, I took a large bite from the apple that I had picked earlier from the apple tree in our garden. While I was eating my apple, my mind drifted. I started thinking about Denmark. My wife and I used to live in Denmark. We bought a house in Bagsværd a suburb located north of Copenhagen. Bagsværd is known for a church designed by Jørn Utzon. Jørn Utzon also designed the Sydney Opera House. The iconic Sydney Opera House was originally budgeted at $7 million but ultimately opened in 1973, coming in at a whopping $102 million. This is 14 times the original budget and a decade later than the original planned date for the grand opening. Kahneman and Tversky referred to a *planning fallacy* in situations where the Base case is founded on unrealistic assumptions that could be easily improved by consulting the statistics of similar cases.

I wondered whether I was a victim of the planning fallacy. Were my timelines to complete the writing of my book *Insight* realistic?

Keeney wrote in his book *Value Focused Thinking* about his collaboration with Ronald Howard. They agreed to collaborate in 1969. The bulk of the writing

---

[40] Swanson's mean is a three-point approximation of a continuous distribution. An alternative weighting scheme for P10:P50:P90 is 25%:50%:25%. However, no matter what choice you make, the approximation progressively worsens if the skewness of the distribution is increased. The mean is higher than the P50 for skewed distribution, and assigning a higher weighting to the P90 provides a better estimate of the mean.

of the nearly 600 pages that make up the book Decision with multiple objectives was done between 1972 and 1976. A four-year period.

Bratvold on the process of writing *Making Good Decisions*: 'The process took "forever". Bratvold and Begg decided to write the book in 2005, finished the draft in 2009, and the book was finally published in 2010. So roughly it had taken them 5 years.

Babak Jafarizadeh told me that it had taken him three years to complete the book *Economic Decision Analysis*. Babak wrote: 'It took me many months in the beginning just to consider the costs and benefits of such a project. Then there is the fact that I wouldn't write anything for weeks or months.'

I completed 120 pages of my Ph. D. thesis in 38 months.

To get a better sense of how long it takes to write a non-fiction book, I made a list of prolific non-fiction authors: Malcolm Gladwell, Nassim Taleb, Adam Grant, Leonard Mlodinow, Margaret Heffernan, Steven Pinker, and Richard Dawkins. I assumed that the authors were writing their books in sequence. I am referring to "Writing Years"[41].

All data are summarised in Table 2.7

	Number of books	First publication year	Last publication year	Period published	Writing years
Malcolm Gladwell	7	2000	2021	21	3.5
Margaret Heffernan	6	2004	2021	17	3.4
Nassim Taleb	5	2001	2019	18	4.5
Adam Grant	4	2014	2021	7	2.3
Leonard Mlodinow	11	2001	2022	21	2.1
Steven Pinker	13	2003	2021	18	1.5
Richard Dawkins	18	1976	2021	45	2.6
Ralph L. Keeney	1	1972	1976	4	4
Reidar Bratvold and Steve Begg	1	2005	2010	5	5
Babak Jafarizadeh	1	2019	2022	3	3
Bart Willigers	1	1995	1999	3.2	3.2

Table 2.7. Assessment of writing years.

---

[41] For all prolific writers, I reduced the book count by one in the calculation of average writing years.

The average number of "writing years" is 2.9. This is almost double the estimated time provided by the *Scientific Publisher*[42] provided: 'Most authors take 1–1.5 years to write their books.'

I started writing in the last week of April, and I have developed a rough plan for what I want to achieve with my writing. I am in the fortunate position that I can spend 20–30 hours a week writing and thinking about my life, my diary, and the insights I have gained in the process. However, if it is really going to take 3 years to finish my book, I would run out of time. In the scenario where I have 1 year of good health, I would be able to finish the book in time. The future is uncertain, and I am not sure whether I have sufficient time to complete this project.

Steve Jobs asked himself 'If today were the last day of my life, would I want to do what I am about to do today?' My answer would be that I would like to finish the first draft of my book before Christmas 2022...and I have achieved that milestone!

4 October 2022: Exploring different options for publishing

BBC Headline: North Korea fires a ballistic missile over Japan

On October 4, 2022, I drew a *strategy table* (Figure 2.15) to assess the options that were available to me. Note that I made this assessment before I was offered a publishing contract.

I thought of four strategies:

> Publishing a series of short stories;
> Publishing a paper;
> Publishing a short book;
> Publishing a comprehensive book.

I also envisaged four decisions:

> Literary agent;
> Writing effort;
> Time horizon;
> Type of publication.

---

[42] I performed the analysis before the publisher made their offer.

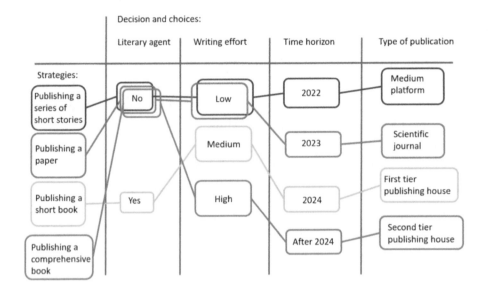

Figure 2.15. Strategy table for exploring the different options for publishing.

I did write a publication that I posted on the Medium platform[43]. I did not write a scientific publication, but I continued to write on my book.

13 October 2022: Feeling of guilt

BBC Headline: Downing Street insists no more U-turns on the mini-budget

The one thing I have struggled with the most over the past months is the fact that I have not been completely honest with my children. I never told them about the real severity of my disease – the fact that there is a tiny chance of me surviving the first two years. I have broken the promise I made to our son – I didn't tell him everything. At this point in time, I simply do not know whether they do know, but they choose to ignore the poor outlook, or whether they genuinely are ignorant about the severeness of the situation.

I also thought about my friends who are suffering from cancer. The role I played in their lives. I questioned whether I had done enough to support them.

---

[43] https://medium.com/

15 November 2022: Preparing for a presentation

BBC Headline: As the 8 billionth child is born, who were the 5th, 6th, and 7th?

My wife and I had an appointment at the hospital. It very much feels like a routine already. My third cycle of chemotherapy is about to start, and I had been given some blood in the morning. We were waiting for the doctor in the waiting room with all these empty seats. We were summoned into a small room, and after a couple of minutes, the doctor appeared. He told us that my platelets were too low to continue the full dose. He suggested reducing the dose to that I had taken in the first cycle.

After we came home, I spoke to a colleague to prepare ourselves for a presentation to be given on the Friday the 18th of November. My colleague gave me the responsibility of delivering this presentation, i.e., getting the slides in order. I went into overdrive to get all the information we needed, in the correct order, into the slide deck. I work until late into the night to get all this done.

1 December 2022: Approval Protocol Complexity tool

BBC Headline: House prices see the biggest fall for two years, says Nationwide

I had arranged to see a colleague for dinner. This was the same person with whom I worked for the presentation on the protocol simplification tool. I ran into him outside the company's office, and he was really excited! Our project was approved by the board. My colleague and I started the development of a tool over a year ago, and it has now been approved for use in all studies undertaken by Biopharma. This was a big, big success for both of us. We have discussed what we should do next. We strategized our next steps and made a list of emails to send the next day. We needed to make some noise to celebrate our success with our broader team. There were approximately 40 team members who all contributed to the development of the tool.

My colleague told me that I looked great, and I felt great. I still struggle to get to grips with the fact that I feel so well and that I might well have a growing tumour in my brain. I told my colleague that I felt like I had just woken up from a really bad dream. Last summer was the hardest period in my life. It was the first time I was confronted with the fragility of life. I was not just worried about myself; I was also deeply worried about my father. Each time I received a message from either my brother or my sister-in-law, especially at unexpected times, my first thought was that Dad had passed away. I was not sure who will die first. I expect it will be me.

My colleague left after he finished his burger, and I stayed for a bit longer and watched some football in the pub. Afterward, I walked to the hotel where I was staying for the night. I checked in and walked to my room. I have read a couple of chapters from Gerd Gigerenzer's book *Reckoning with risk*. I found the book rather difficult to understand. There was a considerable overlap between the topics in Gigerenzer's book and *Insight*, the book I was working on, but I wanted to write a text that was easier to understand. I hoped to would be able to explain this complex material in simpler, more understandable language.

5 December 2022, 27 March 2023, and 26 June 2023: Three revisions of chance of success

The cold facts

I made three assessments on the probability that I would be Progression Free. The facts available to me at the time of making my judgement:

- Base rates Progression Free Survival: December (2022) 58%, March (2023) 38%, June (2023) 25% (these percentages originate from Figure 2.7);
- None of the previous five MRI scans showed cancer growth;
- Even if a tumour was found and I was no longer progression free, I would still have some time to live (Figure 2.7);
- I feel no different now than a year ago. I am not tired and I am not in pain;
- Before the tumour was removed in May 2022, I was completely unaware that a golf-ball-sized tumour had grown in my brain;
- I made all three judgements a couple of days before the scans were made[44], and I would be surprised if my health would significantly change in these two days;
- Over time, there has been a gradual improvement in overall survival (approximately 1% per year[45].

---

[44] I made a judgement on the 2nd of December for a scan made on the 5th of December; I made a judgement on the 24th of March for a scan made on the 27th of December.
[45] Dong et al., 2016; Cioffi et al., 2022.

I am very aware of the difficulty of making an unbiased judgement on the probability that MRI scans will show no sign of new cancer growth. After each MRI scan, I developed three judgements: an Upside case, a Downside case and a Base case (the reader is referred to the section *September 2022 to December 2022: Attempts to draw a decision tree* for the rationale of using these three scenarios, Figure 2.14).

As additional judgements were made, the process was made easier because I could make a new judgement relative to the previous judgements. After each MRI scan, I spent several days pondering, struggling with this assessment but in the end made a judgement between the MRI scan and the outcome.

Judgement of the presence of cancer growth

Table 2.1 lists my personal judgements regarding the probabilities of having no visible tumour on the MRI scans. Note that the assessments I made were all conditional on having no tumour growth detected in the previous scan.

	December 2022	March 2023	June 2023
Upside case	95%	90%	95%
Base case	75%	60%	65%
Downside case	20%	15%	15%

Table 2.1. Probabilities that the scans will show a sign of tumour growth. I have assigned a probability to the Upside, Base, and Downside cases.

I have an MRI scan once every 3 months. As time progresses, the base rate for Progression Free Survival decreases from 58% in December, to 38% in March, and to 25% in June (Figure 2.7).

In December 2022, I was fairly confident that the scan would be clear. In March 2023, I was very nervous, so I made a downward adjustment for both the Base case with fifteen percentage points and the Downside case with five percentage points. I also felt that the upside from December 2022 was a little too optimistic, so I reduced that probability by five percentage points.

The judgement I made for the June 2023 MRI result was made easier by the fact that I had gone through the process several times before and I could create my judgement relative to the judgements I made earlier. For the Upside case, I settled on the same assessment I made in December, i.e., 95%. For the Downside case, I chose the March assessment, i.e., 15%. For the Base case, I judged 65%, i.e., I was less confident in a positive outcome compared with December and slightly more confident than I had been in March.

Estimating the Overall survival

Two key differentiating factors have been identified (Table 2.2): MGMT status[46] and age. I entered survival data from the ten studies into an Excel spreadsheet.

	MGMT status	Age
Balana et al., 2020	Unknown	All ages
Hegi et al., 2005	Known	All ages
Minniti et al., 2009	Unknown	Elderly
Malmström et al., 2012	Known	Elderly
Perry et al., 2017	Known[47]	Elderly
Zur et al., 2020	Unknown	All ages
Zhang et al., 2020	Known	All ages
Stupp et al., 2005	Known	All ages
Stupp et al., 2009	Unknown	All ages
Roa et al., 2015	Unknown	Elderly

Table 2.2. MGMT status and target population.

A series of plots (Figure 2.16) have been made to visualise the Overall Survival projections immediately after the diagnoses (June 2022), after six months (December 2022), after nine months (March 2023), and after twelve months (June 2023). Each plot contains an Upside case (grey), a Downside case (blue) and a Base case (orange). Table 2.3 shows the definitions of these three scenarios. The prognosis is really sensitive to MGMT status and whether the older people are included in the group of patients or not.

---

[46] Butler et al., 2020.

[47] The impact is determined and shown at 12, 18, and 24 months.

	Line colour	MGMT status	Excluding the elderly
Upside case (P90)	Grey	Methylated	Yes
Base case (P50)	Orange	Unmethylated	Yes
Downside case (P10)	Blue	Unmethylated	No

Table 2.3. Three scenarios.

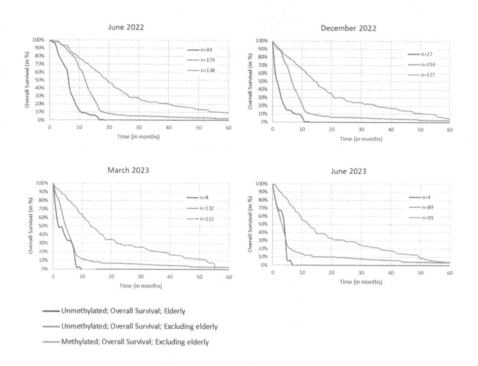

Figure 2.16. Overall Survival at three time points: June 2022, December 2022, March 2023, and June 2023.

Estimating Progression Free Survival

Figure 2.17 (blue symbols) shows how the difference between Overall Survival (OS) and Progression Free Survival (PFS) changes with time.

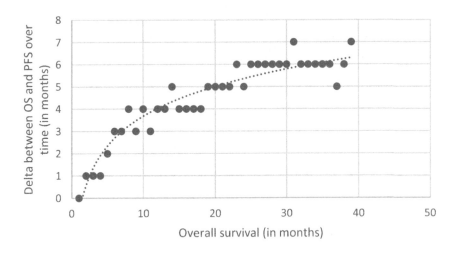

Figure 2.17. The trend of an ever-increasing delta of Overall Survival and Progression Free Survival. OS=Overall Survival, PFS=Progression Free Survival. The equation shown is the fitted curve that describes the trend.

I have fitted the following relationship:

$$PFS = 1.93 \ln(OS) - 0.7521$$

A normal distribution was fitted through the differences between the fitted relationship and the actual observations. This normal distribution has a mean of -0.018 and a standard deviation of 1.16. These statistics were used to define the 80% confidence interval. Because the lower estimate is a negative number, I applied a rather arbitrary cut-off value of 0.1.

Statistics breaking down

As time progresses, fewer and fewer patients remain alive. Consequently, making reliable estimates becomes ever more precarious. This is particularly true for the Downside case. After 12 months, only four patients are Progression Free Survivors. Clearly, one cannot report any reliable statistics on the basis of four patients.

Table 2.4 shows my attempt to obtain more reliable estimates. I used the data plotted in Figure 2.7 and re-baselined[48] this data at 12 months. The results are shown in the column *MGMT status agnostic; Overall Survival; All ages*. Although the method is not perfect, it does preserve the principle of having nine discrete scenarios and a very simple logic to assess the Overall Survival.

		June 2023 data	MGMT status agnostic; Overall Survival; All ages	OS|NT	OS|TG
Upside case	P10	3 (n=99)	1 (n=602)	2	0.1
	P50	12 (n=99)	7 (n=602)	10	4
	P90	61 (n=99)	32 (n=602)	47	12
Base case	P10	1 (n=89)	1 (n=602)	1	0.1
	P50	3 (n=89)	7 (n=602)	5	4
	P90	14 (n=89)	32 (n=602)	23	12
Downside case	P10	1 (n=4)	1 (n=602)	1	0.1
	P50	4 (n=4)	7 (n=602)	6	4
	P90	5 (n=4)	32 (n=602)	19	12

Table 2.4. P10, P50, and P90 estimates of the Upside, Base, and Downside cases. OS=Overall Survival, NT=no tumour (absence of new cancer growth? is "Yes") and TG=tumour growth (absence of new cancer growth? is "No"). OS|NT = Overall Survival given that no tumour is found.

Time to life as time moves on

We can now estimate Overall Survival time in a logical framework. A probability tree has been developed (see section *September 2022 to December 2022: Attempts to draw a decision tree*, Figure 2.14). All probabilities have been defined (see sections *September 2022 to December 2022: Attempts to draw a decision tree* and *Judgement on the presence of cancer growth*). Finally, the length of Overall Survival is shown in table 2.5.

---

[48] I achieve this by first removing all percentages in the first year. Taking the Progression Free percentage at month i divided by the Progression Free percentage at month $i = 1$ (i.e., Progression Free percentage in month 12 originally). I applied this logic to all remaining periods.

		June 2022	December 2022		March 2023		June 2023	
		OS	OS|NT	OS|TG	OS|NT	OS|TG	OS|NT	OS|TG
Upside case	P10	7	2	0.1	3	0.1	2	0.1
	P50	20	15	3	13	3	10	4
	P90	57	54	9	53	9	47	12
Base case	P10	6	3	0.1	1	0.1	1	0.1
	P50	13	7	3	5	3	5	4
	P90	19	14	9	12	9	23	12
Downside case	P10	3	1	0.1	1	0.1	1	0.1
	P50	7	3*	3	3*	3	6	4
	P90	11	9	9	9*	9	19	12

Table 2.5. P10, P50, and P90 estimates of the Upside, Base, and Downside cases. OS=Overall Survival, NT=no tumour (absence of new cancer growth? is "Yes") and TG=tumour growth (absence of new cancer growth? is "No"). OS|NT = Overall Survival given that no tumour is found. * The original estimate was 2, ** The original estimate was 8.

Please note that in the Overall Survival numbers in the Downside case in March for the Tumour Growth scenario were actually higher than those for the No Tumour scenario. Given that the No Tumour scenario was based on eight patients, I deemed the Tumour Growth scenario more representative. Hence, I used those numbers for both scenarios in the probability tree, as shown in Figure 2.19[49].

Over the last 9 months, my median Overall Survival time has changed between 7 months in December, 9 months in March, and 5 months in June[50]. However, as time passes, the actual calendar date moves forward. At the time of writing (June 29, 2023), my expected death is in November 2023. Given that these distributions are highly skewed, the latest estimate for the mean Overall Survival time is twice as long as the median of 10 months. Therefore, according to the mean Overall Survival time I would be still alive in April 2024.

---

[49] I could have simplified the probability tree, but I chose not to do so for consistency reasons. In June 2023, for example, I developed different estimates for these scenarios.
[50] I developed the probability tree after the MRI scan was performed in September 2022; therefore, I did not make a probability assessment for the September MRI scan.

Final thoughts on modelling survival times

Collapsing width of the confidence interval

The rationale behind the three scenarios; Upside case, Base case and Downside case, was to create three outcomes that were significantly different. An alternative approach is to calculate the confidence intervals and report the P10 and P90 values. However, the issue with this approach is that the confidence intervals are very narrow. The width of the confidence interval is controlled by the number of observations. The higher the number of observations, the narrower the confidence interval. The more data, the smoother the curves. There is a trade-off between curve smoothness and shrinking confidence intervals. This trade-off is illustrated in Figure 2.18. The figure illustrates that the blue lines based on 1172 patients are much smoother than the orange lines based on 44 patients. The figure also shows that the distance between the two dashed lines is much smaller for the set of blue lines than for the set of orange lines.

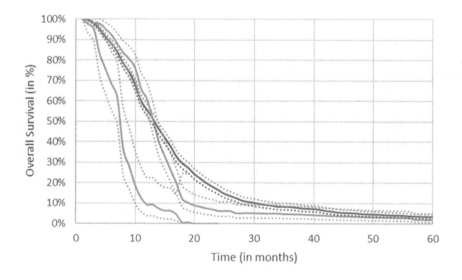

Figure 2.18. Relationship between the number of observations and the width of the confidence interval.

I inserted the judgements that I made in late February – early March 2023 before I met with my doctor into the probability tree, as shown in Figure 2.19, and a cumulative probability plot, as shown in Figure 2.20.

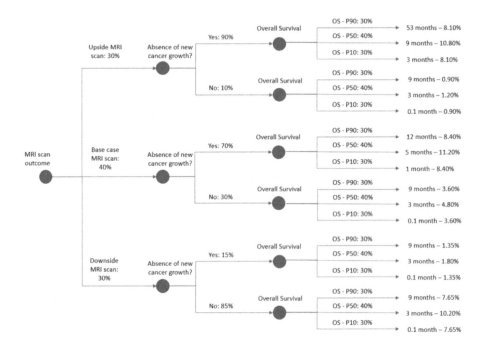

Figure 2.19. Probability tree populated with the estimated outcomes and probabilities. Probabilities I assigned before I had the meeting with my doctor (prior) in March 2023. OS = Overall Survival.

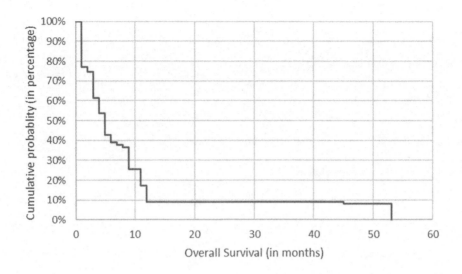

Figure 2.20. Cumulative probability plot of overall survival before meeting with my doctor (prior) in March 2023.

This probability tree has a P50 Overall Survival of 9 months and an expected Overall Survival of 10 months. The overall P50 was obtained by sorting all scenarios in decreasing order of Overall Survival, subsequently calculating the cumulative probabilities, and finally reading the cumulative probability at 50%.

I made this assessment on the morning of March 24, the day I received the results of my MRI scan. It was good news: no new growth was detected in the MRI scan. I was so happy! Although I was not surprised by this outcome as I had assigned a probability of 70% that I would be progression free, it was still a big relief to me, my wife, my family, and my close friends.

I have updated my probability tree. As the scan was a week old, I was not completely sure whether there was still any visible sign of the tumour. Therefore, I did not set the probabilities at 100%. Figure 2.21 shows the updated tree immediately after I received the new information.

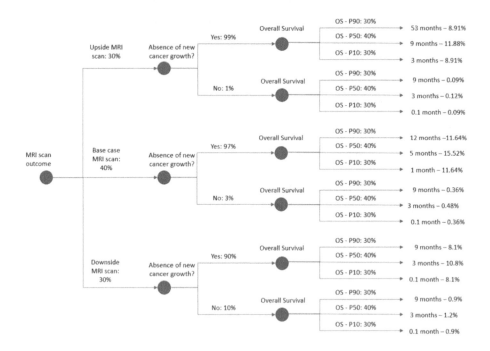

Figure 2.21. The posterior probability tree is populated with estimated outcomes and probabilities. The probabilities I assigned after I had a meeting with my doctor in March 2023.

Although I was delighted with the scan result, upon analysing the data, I concluded that little had changed. The median value was still 9 months, and the mean value increased from 1 month to 11 months. I must admit that I was somewhat disappointed; I had expected to see a larger movement.

Simplification of the real world

The fact that the P50 estimate hardly changed after we updated the probabilities in the probability tree is an artefact of the modelling approach we adopted. We have simplified the continuous distribution into a series of discrete scenarios. Every mathematical model is a simplification of the real world, and there are many trade-offs to consider. In this case, it is much easier, in fact infinitely easier, for the human mind to consider a set of discrete scenarios rather than a continuous distribution (which encompasses an infinite number of scenarios).

Clearly, one could add more and more probability-weighted percentages to improve the reality of the model. Such an approach would add to the workload, and it is not obvious when to stop this refinement process. On the one hand, more points are always better, but there is a decreasing incremental improvement with each point added.

17 January 2023: The box on the attic

BBC Headline: Madonna announces a Career-spanning greatest hits tour

Gone are the days when the noise was deafening. The glass windowpanes vibrated to their breaking point. The noise kept me awake during the night. There were two types of noise: a high-pitch sound and a low-base sound. The vibration of the base caused every glass, piece of cutlery, and plate in the kitchen to rattle. The low-frequency sound was a constant in my life for many months. It never went away, and at times I was convinced it was there to stay. The high-pitch sound came in waves. It was overwhelming. I was desperate trying to reduce the volume of the noise and simply not being able to do so. I was struggling to contain these screams, these vivid visions, and this anxiety.

It has taken me over 8 months, but now I have finally been able to put all of these noises in a box. I placed this box in the attic. The box contains all my anxiety about dying. Now I feel I can open it up and close it again as I wish. When I open the box and look inside, I see visions of myself lying on my deathbed. I am unable to move, and it looks as if I am asleep. I am dying in my vision but seem to have no suffering or pain. Once I have looked at this vision for a while, I can close the box, put down the lid, lock it, and get on with my life.

2 February 2023: Treatment in the USA or the UK

BBC Headline: Over-50s at work: 'You feel your usefulness has passed'

The previous week, I had spoken to a former colleague of mine. After a reorganisation, she left the company, but we remained in contact. We spoke about my illness and how I was treated in the UK. She suggested that I approach an oncology colleague based in the USA. The philosophy of treating patients in the USA is very different from that in the UK.

Today, I received an email from a colleague who specialises in oncology and has a large network in the oncologist's community. In her email, she gave me the contact details of a couple of doctors in New York. I followed a link that I found on the website. I looked at the headshot picture and read that the doctor was a German who had moved to the USA a couple of decades ago.

I was in the kitchen in the process of making a cup-a-soup sunken in deep thoughts, reflecting on this German doctor. I suddenly realised that I could not hear my wife on the telephone – my wife had been on the phone most in the morning. I walked up to her little office, which is located next to the kitchen. I had read the German doctor's profile half an hour ago and realised that I could not take this any further without having discussed the matter with my dear wife.

The main difference between the UK and the USA is that in the USA, glioblastoma patients are often treated with Avastin. Avastin has a very different side effect profile than Temozolomide, the drug that has been used in my treatment. Although I had suffered little to virtually no side effects from Temozolomide (TMZ), it is unknown to me nor any of the medical experts who are treating me how my body would react if I were to switch to Avastin. However, more importantly, neither my wife nor I had seen any evidence of any significant differences in mortality rates.

My wife and I discussed our family's Quality of Life. If I were to be treated in the USA, it was clear to both of us that that decision would have a negative impact on my family's Quality of Life. I would have to travel to the USA, which would require making travel plans and planning for hospital visits; we also had to book hotel rooms, arrange for taxi rides, etc. It would severely disrupt our current family life. In addition, there are cost implications – treatment was not going to be cheap.

Going through this list of issues, we concluded that staying at my current hospital was the preferred option.

I went back upstairs to my office and changed into my cycle gear. The only thing I could fully control was where my next bike ride would take me. Once I into my cycle gear, I went down the stairs where I ran into my wife. My wife had finished my cup-a-soup and was taking it to my office. She said something along the lines of "…I did not want to sound too negative…"

Decision Quality in Action

Although it might not be obvious to the casual reader, I used Decision Quality to decide. I went through all six elements of good decision practises:

1. Frame: Seek an alternative hospital for further treatment
2. Values: Quality of Life
3. Alternatives: Current hospital or a US hospital (e.g., New York)
4. Information: There is no significant extension of life in the USA compared with the UK. Treatment in the USA is expensive, and the side effects of Avastin are unknown
5. Reasoning: Logical deduction that our Quality of Life would be reduced
6. Commitment to action: I involved my wife in the discussion

I decided to stay with the current hospital for now.

28 February 2023: Finished chemotherapy

BBC Headline: Carbon capture: What is it and how does it fight climate change?

I finished my sixth and final chemotherapy cycle yesterday. I slept very poorly last night. I did not make a connection between chemotherapy and lying awake until I had been awake for several hours. I was not feeling ill, had no nausea whatsoever, and was feeling completely fine. Strange this chemotherapy! I did a lot of thinking about my book and how to progress and finalise it. I also thought about the children – how would my disease impact them over the coming months?

7 March 2023: The creative process of writing a book

BBC Headline: How many people cross the Channel in small boats and where do they come from?

It has taken me over a year to write this book. During this time, I used the same creative process many times. Once I identified a topic that I deemed relevant to my book, I went through a four-step process, as shown in Figure 2.22. The four steps are:

1. Saturation: I researched the topic by reading widely and deeply. At some point, I stopped collecting information and started to organize, sort, and evaluate this information.
2. Incubation: I would be mulling over the information that I had collected. What should the outline look like, which structure would make sense to the reader, and how to prioritise the information? This process would take a couple of days (and nights), often unconsciously.

3. Illumination: I would experience typical "ah-ha" moments when suddenly bits of information fell into place and I would become conscious of an even bigger picture.
4. Writing: I would write down a draft, re-read it, and rewrite the text.

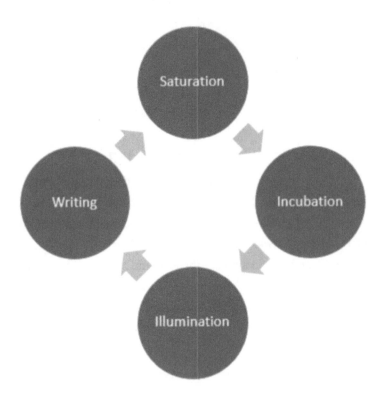

Figure 2.22. The creative process of writing.

As I was writing, I had multiple cycles operating in my brain. So, while I was reading up on one topic, I was unconsciously reflecting on another topic. Likewise, I was writing one chapter when I suddenly experienced an "ah-ha" moment about a completely different topic.

My wife, son, and I drove up north to meet our daughter and my mother-in-law for lunch. It was really good to see both of them! The children started to tease each other. They must have missed each other. I felt very grateful to see them again and to have the opportunity to share a meal with them.

22 March 2023: Mum's and Dad's bizarre birthdays

BBC Headline: UN warns against "vampiric" global water use

I travelled to the Netherlands to visit my parents and attend their birthdays. Mum will turn 80 years old this year, Dad will turn 81 years old this year. The two birthday parties are a really bizarre experience for me. This might well be the last time I meet my parents' friends and my uncles and aunts. Although all of them are two to three decades older than me, it is highly likely that I will be the first or perhaps the second one to die. Me and Mum's sister are at the highest risk of dying. Mum's sister was diagnosed with pancreatic cancer last December. I sat next to her during Mum's party, and we shared our experiences – both of us are living from day to day.

The paper on elicitation that was originally submitted to the *New England Journal of Medicine* back in May has officially been accepted by the journal *Advances in Therapy*. The manuscript was submitted four times. Each time we spent time revising the manuscript before we resubmitted an updated version, we have spent so much time and effort on getting our article published.

5 April 2023: No cancer growth in my skull!

BBC Headline: Trump charged: One thing his day in court tells us

Great news! No new cancer growth in my skull. I am so incredible relieved. I struggled to wrap my head around the news that my doctor gave me – I am so grateful.

After we received this fantastic news, we followed the advice from my doctor: we walked into Trailfinders and picked up some materials on Africa and Canada. After some discussions, we decided that southern or eastern Africa was our preference, and eventually, we decided to go to Tanzania!

22 April 2023: Objective network for writing insights

As time progressed and my brain tumour remained under control, I became more relaxed about my health. In March 2023, I finished my second draft of *Insight* and started collecting information on how to get my book published. I had approached several publishers and agents, and I had spoken to people who had published books. On the 22nd of April, I received an email that a scientific publisher had accepted my book proposal.

Rather than simply accepting this offer, I performed some analysis: 1) I drew an objective network and 2) I executed a weighted ranking exercise on the options available to me[51].

Objective network Insight

While I was writing, I had some thoughts about what I wanted to achieve with my writing, but I never took the time to put those thoughts down in a structured way. Acceptance of the manuscript by a *Scientific Publisher* was the trigger to do so.

I started by copying the personal objective network that I had already developed. I noticed that in the *Insight* project, I was addressing identical strategic objectives as I had previously defined in my personal objective network[52]. I have relabelled strategic objectives to fundamental objectives as we are dealing with a much narrower, more specific, decision problem.

The most important objective for me is to maximise the impact of my book *Insight*. I believe this can be achieved by creating a book that is easy to read and affordable so that it can sell many copies (either physical or digitally). In addition, I believe that the book can strengthen my family relationships, create new opportunities, and provide personal monetary benefits.

Readability is determined by an engaging writing style, which ensures that the book is well structured (sign posted) and that the text is free from grammar and spelling errors. My ambition for this book is to cover all topics that are of relevance to decision-making and discuss all statistical concepts needed to understand oncology trials. The book must be free of any conceptual errors.

Accessibility is largely determined by the publisher's choice. The publisher needs a brand to reach as many readers as possible and must set a price as low as possible. The contract also covers the details of the renumeration of the publishing author.

Ultimately, all these objectives translate into my fundamental objective of maximising happiness. The final objective network is shown in Figure 2.23.

---

[51] The reader is referred to section "10 June2023: Selection of publisher". I accepted the offer by the second publisher who was willing to publish *Insight*.

[52] I was expecting that some strategic objectives were not relevant because the scope is much narrower than the situation I analysed when I was drawing my objective network.

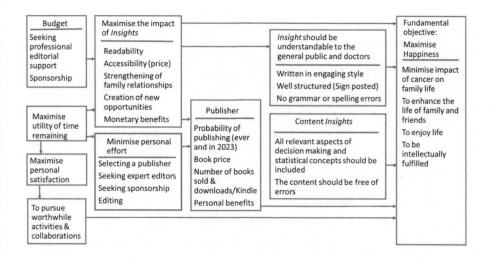

Figure 2.23. Objective network for publishing my book.

The objective of section *10 June 2023: Selecting a publisher* is much more specific. This section focuses on one aspect of my objective network – the selection of a publisher. The decision context "finding the right publisher" has become the fundamental objective. Many objectives listed in Figure 2.23 are irrelevant. For example, the "readability of the book" bears no relation to the publisher I select. The five considerations are relevant: Book revenue, probability of publishing in 2024, number of downloads/Kindle, personal benefit, and personal effort.

24 April 2023: A year has passed since the tumour was found

BBC Headline: Local elections 2023: How sewage topped the political agenda

I have a mailing list of the colleagues I feel closest to. Today, I mailed this email that was several weeks overdue:

Dear Friends,

I wanted you to know that there were no signs of cancer growth in the latest MRI scan. I was so relieved.

This week, it has been a year since the tumour was discovered.

Cheers,

Bart

10 June 2023: Selecting the publisher

There are three aspects that are really important to me in choosing the optimal route of getting *Insight* published: number of copies sold, book price, and probability of getting the book published. I am much less concerned about my personal gain in the project, nor the amount of personal effort required to get it published.

I settled on five decision criteria (Table 2.7). I assigned a relative score using the principles described in the *Multi-Criteria Decision Analysis*[53] section.

Criteria	Raw weights	Weights
Number of books/Kindle /downloads sold	6	27.27%*
Book price	6	27.27%
Probability of publication in 2024	6	27.27%
Personal benefit	3	13.64%
Personal effort	1	4.55%
Total:	22	

Table 2.7. Weighting of the decision criteria * 6/22=27.27%

Table 2.8 summarises the facts I gathered and the judgements I made.

I consider the *number of copies of books and digital downloads* either from the publisher's website or through Kindle ultimately driven by the strength of the publisher's brand. I refer to this as a *premium brand*. I assigned a score of one to the Premium Brand. I do not have a personal brand. "Bart Willigers" is not a household name. Although I have published over 50 scientific papers, many of those papers were published years ago and had little impact, if any, on the

---

[53] This chapter can be found in Part 3 of the book.

public. Hence, I scored myself a 0.001, i.e., for every thousand copies sold by the Premium Brand, I will sell a single copy on my own. I estimated that Austin Macauley Publishers would sell as many copies as a scientific publisher with open access. I scored both options with a 0.6. However, a scientific publisher without open access has a much lower score. I allocated a score of 0.2 to this option. The *Agency*[54] option is scored with a 0.5.

The book price should be as low as possible to ensure that as many readers as possible have access to the book. Hardback books retail for £20 to £35, softback books retail for £9 to £15. As I am doing a relative scoring, I scored 1 for all book options except Scientific Publisher. Scientific Publishers are sold at a premium. Scientific Publisher with open access and Scientific Publisher without open access I scored 0.8 and 0.3, respectively.

I would like to maximise the *Probability to publish in 2024.* I want to publish as soon as possible – it is essential to me to get the book read by people. The sure route for publishing in 2023–2024 is by either publishing independently, Scientific Publisher, with or without open access, or Austin Macauley Publishers. Hence, I gave these options a score of 1. Premium Brand represents any large publisher. Many of them will only accept manuscripts from agents or they have indicated on their websites that they do not have no spare capacity to review new manuscripts. I assigned a score of 0.2 to Premium Brand and a score of 0.4 to Agency.

There is a second probability that needs to be assessed. Namely, the probability that the manuscript will ever get published – *Probability to publish.* These two probabilities refer to different things. The first probability is derived from the value system. To me, it is essential that the book be published as soon as possible. At this point in time, June 2023, I believe that there is a high likelihood that I will die in a year's time. The second probability refers to the chance of success of the book, i.e., the probability that this book will be released in the future. I am worried that once I am gone, there will be no one who will push this project to completion.

I believe that *personal benefit* is maximised if I release the book independently, so I gave that option a score of 1. Scientific Publisher is willing to pay a flat fee with little upside. I gave Scientific Publisher a score of 0.1. Austin Macauley Publishers has offered a percentage of the net profit from book

---

[54] There are many sites available to find a literary agent, e.g., https://jerichowriters.com/non-fiction-how-to-find-a-literary-agent-for-non-fiction/

sales. I gave the others a lower score than Austin Macauley Publishers but significantly higher than Scientific Publisher. I assigned scores of 0.8, 0.7, and 0.5 to Austin Macauley Publishers, Premium Brand, and Agency, respectively.

Personal effort consists of the effort to find a publisher or agent and the effort required in publishing the book. In my judgement, there will be a lot of effort required to get the book in the correct format if I choose the independent route. I also expect that I would have to invest much time and effort when I opt for the Premium Brand or Agency option to find a party interested in publishing the manuscript.

	Independent	Scientific Publisher open access	Scientific Publisher without open access	Austin Macauley Publishers	Premium Brand	Agency
Raw scores:						
Number of books/downloads/Kindle sold	0.0001	0.6	0.2	0.6	1	0.5
Book price:	1	0.8	0.3	1	1	1
Probability to publish in 2024	1	1	1	1	0.2	0.4
Personal benefit	1	0.1	0.1	0.8	0.7	0.5
Personal effort	0.6	0.8	0.8	0.9	0.2	0.2
Normalised scores:						
Number of books/downloads/Kindle sold	0	0.207*	0.069	0.207	0.345	0.172
Book price	0.196	0.157	0.059	0.196	0.196	0.196
Probability to publish in 2024	0.217	0.217	0.217	0.217	0.043	0.087
Personal benefit	0.313	0.031	0.031	0.25	0.219	0.156

Personal effort	0.171	0.229	0.229	0.257	0.057	0.057
Probability score:						
Probability to publish	1	1	1	1	0.4	0.8

Table 2.8. Scoring of publishing alternatives.

$$* \ 0.207 \ = 0.6/(0.0001 + 0.6 + 0.2 + 0.6 + 1 + 0.5)$$

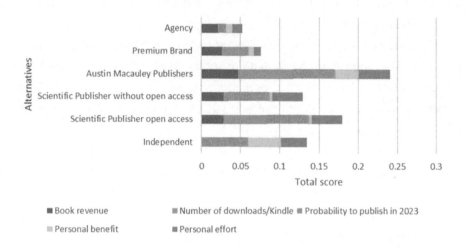

Figure 2.24. Assessment of alternative publication routes.

I summed the normalised score and multiplied this score by the *Probability to publish*. Figure 2.24 shows the results of my assessment. At the time, I executed the scoring, and the manuscript had been accepted by two publishers: Scientific Publisher and Austin Macauley Publishers. As Austin Macauley Publishers yielded the highest score, I signed their contract.

4 July 2023: The return of the tumour

BBC Headline: Wimbledon 2023: Eight-time champion Roger Federer is honoured in Centre Court ceremony

'I had learned a couple of basic rules. The first detailed statistics are for research halls, not hospital rooms. Rather than saying, "Median survival is eleven months" or "You have a ninety-five percent chance of being dead in two years," I'd say "Most patients live many months to a couple of years." This was, to me, a more honest description.

Paul Kalanithi in *When Breath Becomes Air*

Whilst the Americans were waking up for a day to celebrate Independence Day, the 4th of July, I was told by my doctor that my tumour had started to grow again. Now the tumour had started growing again, I was no longer Progression Free and I was given 6 months to life. According to my estimation, I have a median Overall Survival time of 4 months and an average of slightly over 5 months Overall Survival time[55].

The following day at 11:45, the doctor called. The doctor had been in their usual Thursday morning meeting with the other doctors from the medical team. He advised me to have a second operation…and he was not impressed by our vacation plans. I learned that it not advisable to travel to Tanzania for a safari with a growing brain tumour in your head.

We ignored the doctor's advice and boarded a plane to Tanzania the following Friday. Tanzania was FANTASTIC! Going to Tanzania was the best decision we have made since I was diagnosed with a brain tumour. Admittedly I am a little nervous whether this decision will lead to an undesirable outcome as this trip has delayed surgery for 16 days. However, if my tumour is so aggressive that the pre-operation scan will change the surgeon's view on the operation, my life will end soon anyway…

27 July 2023: Meeting the surgeon

BBC Headline: Hollywood writers fear losing their work to AI

This morning, I spent an hour drafting a list of givens, uncertainties, and decisions.

The results are shown in Table 2.6. These issues will form the basis of our discussions with the medical team today and tomorrow.

---

[55] $0.3*12 + 0.4*4 + 0.3*0.1 = 5.23$ months to death

Issues
Givens

Tumour regrowth visible on MRI scan

Prognosis: 6 months until death after the first sign of cancer regrowth

TMZ is no longer effective

The first operation was successfully completed

No significant reduction in QoL using radiation and TMZ

Bart is physically fit and mentally strong

Large uncertainties will persist for a long time (survival, QoL)

The hospital is world class

Maggies/MacMillan support for me, my wife, and our children

Uncertainties to us (but givens to the medical team)

What is the treatment plan (operation, radiation, chemo)?

How much risk is associated with a second operation?

How much less effective is the new chemotherapy compared with TMZ?

Is treatment with Avastin a possibility?

Are there clinical trials for which Bart would qualify?

Uncertainties that persist (to both the medical team and us)

When will we find new cancer growth (a third occurrence)?

What is the speed of cancer growth (a third occurrence)?

Our decisions for now (what is in our control)

Should we approve a second operation?

If Avastin could be used, would we be willing to spend the money?

Choose a clinical trial

Healthy lifestyle choices

Prioritisation of tasks (family, writing, work)

Our decisions for later (what is in our control)

Preparation for my funeral

Retrieval driving licence

Table 2.6. Listing of givens, uncertainties, and decisions.

My wife and I spoke to the surgeon in the afternoon. He gave a clear explanation on the pros and cons of the operation. Apparently, the biggest risk of the operation is an infection of the wound[56]. The risk of damaging brain tissue was not worrying the surgeon, i.e., that risk was the same as during the first operation.

---

[56] I did not ask him for a probability as the surgeon was not very enthusiastic given the probabilities of certain events happening last year. I did not ask him for the probability. However, given that he mentioned this risk and that the risk for an infection doubled, I estimate this risk to be about 10%.

28 July 2023: Gathering information for a decision tree

BBC Headline: Climate change: July set to be world's warmest month on record

We arranged a second meeting with a representative from the medical team. At the end of this meeting, I had gathered all the information I needed to draw a decision tree.

The decision tree is shown in Figure 2.25. I decided to undergo the operation. The key factors that I considered were:

- Operation might not be an option in the future;
- An operation does not prevent the use of chemotherapy and radiation therapy at a later date;
- This decision has no impact on my participation in subsequent clinical studies;
- I am happy to follow the advice of my medical team during subsequent treatment and;
- The outcome of a pre-operation MRI scan is out of my control, so there is no need for me to worry about this scan.

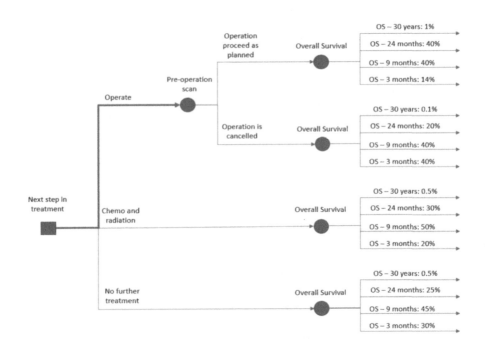

Figure 2.25. The decision tree that I used in my decision to perform the second operation.

31 July 2023: Scenario planning

BBC Headline: When will it stop raining and the summer improve?

This morning, I woke up sweating. Over the last year, my mind has been completely occupied by my disease and the associated shortening of my expected life span. I had come to grips with the fact that my remaining life had been reduced to a couple of years. I had become used to the visions of a brain tumour gradually filling my skull, the grief of my family and friends, and me cremation ceremony.

What I hadn't contemplated was a scenario in which I would still be alive in thirty years. What would I do in that case? How would I cope with all those years? I woke up sweating because I was not prepared for that scenario. I felt that I had been blinded for this – admittedly very unlikely – outcome.

The goal of *Scenario planning* is to develop different perspectives on how the world can ultimately turn out. The objective of Scenario planning is to develop internally consistent scenarios that trigger different sets of decisions. One should resist the temptation to assign probabilities to any specific scenario.

The trends are listed in Table 2.7, and the uncertainties are listed in Table 2.8. A description of the three scenarios of different of Overall Survival are shown in Table 2.9.

Trends:	Description:
Future well-being	I am anxious about my future mental and physical health. I consider it likely that I have a year left, and I want to make the time remaining worthwhile.
Increasing risk of chronic disease with age	As with all human beings, my personal risk of contracting chronic diseases will increase as I get older.
Death	The only certainty we have is that 1 day we will die.
Pharmaceutical companies are committed to oncology	The fact that large investments are made in oncology suggests that a cure for cancer is no longer deemed impossible.
Cancer as a chronic disease	Breast and prostate cancers are chronic diseases, especially when diagnosed early.
24 years passed without any novel treatment	TMZ was approved for medical use in 1999. This was the last breakthrough treatment for brain tumours.

Overall Survival rate is improving	Improvement in radiation treatments has led to an increase, with a couple of percentile points per year, in Overall Survival.
Less effective treatment	TMZ is currently the most effective treatment, also the next radiation treatment will be at a lower dose – so the next round of treatment will be less effective.
Genomics data, machine learning, and artificial intelligence	Recently, several papers have been published on genomics data[57]. This, along with the ever-increasing power of machine learning and artificial intelligence, might lead to a future cure of brain tumour.

Table 2.7. Trends.

Uncertainties:	Description:
Overall Survival	My Overall Survival is estimated at 12 months (at the end of July 2023)
Cognitive abilities	In my judgement, the probability that a complication occurs during the operation is 15%.
Cure of brain tumours	In my judgement, the probability that a cure will be found in the next decade is negligible – smaller than 1%.

Table 2.8. Uncertainties.

Scenarios:	Description:
Quick ending	After brain surgery, I do not fully recover, and my cognitive abilities are compromised. I do not go back to work, but I still perform some physical exercise and try to publish *Insight*. I prepare for my funeral.
One healthy year	I have a single healthy year left. I give my family and friends the opportunity to get on with their lives. Our daughter enjoys her year abroad, our son gets a good set of exam results, and my wife plans to return to Scotland. I will also support my brother, my parents, and my friends to the best of my ability. I will return to work and publish *Insight*.
Long life	I will be cured of my brain tumour within a decade. I will reach the grand age of 80 years. My wife and I will move to Scotland in two years, and we will travel the world. I will ensure that I have a good

---

[57] E.g., Gusev *et al.*, 2018.

	relationship with both my children. I will find a different occupation. *Insight* will become a bestseller; I will make a name for myself and give lectures on decision analysis. I retrieve my driving licence

Table 2.9. Scenarios.

17 August 2023: Past decisions and their outcomes

BBC headline: Sarina Wiegman[58]: FA says any approaches would be "100% rejected"

I have been reflecting on the two hardest decisions I have made in my life. The decision to give up geology and to relocate from Scotland to England. The common factor in these two decisions is that both involved an impossible trade-off.

I gave up geology in 2000. Before I stopped being a geologist, I had finished my Ph.D. course and started my first postdoctoral research. At the time, the job prospects for geologists were horrendous – metal prices and oil prices were both at rock bottom, and I perceived that the uncertainty of employment in academia was simply too large. Despite these facts, I really loved my job. I had so much joy while being a geologist. Poor job prospects were nothing new. The job market has always been volatile, going through cycles of boom and bust. Had I remained single, there would have been no issue, but I started seeing a girl. This girl became my wife a couple of years later, and we started talking about raising a family. Therefore, I felt it was time to pack in my geology "hobby" and find a well-paid real job. Ultimately, I ended up being enrolled in an MBA programme in the Netherlands – Nyenrode University. The trade-offs were between my personal strategy objective "Maximise Happiness"[59] and "Minimise the burden I place on my family"[60]. At the time "financial well-being" trumped "intellectual fulfilment". However, even after all these years, I am still a geologist at heart. Geology fulfilled my scientific curiosity.

---

[58] Sarina is a childhood friend of a friend of mine.

[59] I recognised three elements to "Maximise Happiness". The second one "To be intellectually fulfilled" is the objective that I failed to achieve.

[60] I recognised that there are three elements to "Minimise the burden I place on my family". The second one "Maximise financial well-being" is the objective that I prioritised.

The second difficult decision was relocation from Scotland to England. We had a really nice life in Scotland. I suspect that Scotland is the only place where I ever felt truly happy. As my strategic objective is "Maximise Happiness", moving to England was a mistake. Not only did I prefer the Scottish lifestyle we had, but I also believe that my family did so too. The reason for moving to England was to advance my career. I wanted to "Maximise financial well-being". At the time, I was facing redundancy. Shell had acquired my previous employer, and all of us were literally on the firing line. There was massive uncertainty regarding the economy in northeast Scotland, and I was not ready for a massive cut in salary. Visions of being unemployed were haunting me. Scotland's romance would have worn off very quickly on me. Therefore, when a pharmaceutical company offered me a contract, I grabbed the opportunity.

The concept of "even swaps"[61] might sound appealing in theory, but in practise, it is very difficult to apply.

These two decisions made me wonder "what if" – "what if" I pursued my career in geology for a little while longer?– "what if" I decided to stay in Scotland? There are still geologists working as geologists, and there are still people living in the village where we used to live. As time progresses, it becomes increasingly difficult to imagine how life could have turned out...

The reason why I discussed these two decisions in detail is to show that even a decision analyst is sometimes struggling to make the right decision.

29 August 2023: Waking up with no loss of cognition

BBC headline: People stranded as UK flight disruption "set to last days"

I had my second brain surgery on the 21st of August 2023. Like the previous operation, I reported at reception at 7:00 am Monday morning and like the first time, I was booked in for the second slot scheduled for the afternoon. This meant that I had a long wait ahead of me. When I spoke to the surgeon in the morning, he told me that for the patient, the operation was over in an instant. After the operation, the patient simply wakes up completely oblivious to the amount of time that has passed. For the medical team responsible for the operation, the

---

[61] The concept of sacrificing time for money (how much money will you be willing to spend to get the project finished a month earlier?) or Quality of Life for Quantity of Life (how much is an additional one-year be worth to you if your Quality of Life during that year is halved?).

operation lasts about 10 h. The team must align the head with the MRI scan imagery, open the skull, remove the cancerous growth, and finally stitch the wound back together. For the family, the operation takes for ever – time slows right down – and their wait seems to last for an eternity…

Just before 14:00, I found myself dressed in an operation gown and lying on a bed that was pushed around the hospital on its way to the operation theatre. I remember being pushed into the operating theatre just before I fell into deep sleep.

When I regained consciousness, I instantly knew that the operation had been successful. I felt the same as before the operation – I had lost none of my cognitive abilities. I felt delighted!

I spent two nights in the hospital. During the first night, I struggled to sleep because of all the beeping sounds of various alarms going off around the various wards. One of these sounds came from a blood pressure metre. As it turned out, these measuring devices were given to the ward several years ago, and one of the nurses told me that the alarm sounds were related to low battery power. I was kept awake by an alarm due to poor battery performance! This sounded like an example of *Story Bias*.

Story Bias is the notion that human beings tend to simplify life into a basic narrative. One thing leads smoothly and logically to the next. Story Bias removes the notion of random events. Although life is a sequence of random events – one arbitrary event followed by the next – this is not what we remember about our lives. It feels that certain events are meant to happen to us; we are predestined to a series of logical events[62].

At night, in a hospital ward, one expects a noisy scene. The groans of patients, the beeping of machines, and chatting nurses are all sounds that are expected. The sound of a senseless alarm fits into this nightly scene. What baffles me is that no one has noticed that the sounding of this alarm simply does not

---

[62] Another example of Story Bias is shown in the 1998 film *Sliding Doors*. Sliding doors tells a story about a young woman, called Helen, who rushes out to catch a train when two realities split into two scenarios. In one scene, she gets on the train and comes home to find her boyfriend in bed with another woman. In the second, she misses the train and arrives after the woman has left. In the first scenario, Helen dumps her boyfriend, finds a new man, and gradually improves her life. In the second, she becomes suspicious of her boyfriend's fidelity and becomes miserable.

make any sense – even after a week of contemplation, I still cannot think of any purpose for this alarm.

The timing of my operation and our daughter's travel plans could not have been worse. I had my operation on Monday evening, and our daughter set off on Thursday morning; she booked a very early flight. Our daughter had planned to move abroad for a year to study.

On Saturday morning, my wife and son would follow our daughter. Apart from the necessary planning for my family, we also arranged for my brother and his wife to come over for the weekend to look after me. The three of us had a lovely weekend – we went for a couple of car drives, had a couple of pints at two local pubs, attended a village party, and prepared some nice meals.

4 September 2023: Losing control of your life

BBC headline: New tech boosts Dutch drive for sustainable farming

Over the weekend, I started reading *Being Mortal* by Atul Gawande. One of the key observations in his book is that older people become deeply unhappy once they move into a retirement home. The main reason for this unhappiness is a sudden loss of freedom to choose. Upon moving into a retirement home, people invariably lose their independence in decision making. The retirement home decides what time to get up in the morning, what time to have breakfast, when you should take your medication, etc. – people lose their right to decide. Typically, it is children of elderly parents who have decided that their parents can no longer live independently. A sequence of events typically preceded this decision: repeated falls, memory loss, driving accidents, or a combination of these. Children face a stark trade-off between "safety" and "the wish of (one of) their parents to be independent".

In his book, Atul refers to a study executed by Laura Carstensen[63], in which she compared the views of adult men aged between 23 and 66. Some men were terminally ill with HIV/AIDS. She concluded that the preferences of terminally ill patients converged to the outlook of elderly people, i.e., their views became fully aligned regardless of their age.

Like these HIV/AIDS patients, my outlook is equally dark. My doctor told me that I will not grow old. Recently, I have been reflecting on my life since I was diagnosed with a brain tumour. I believe that my biggest personal

---

[63] Carstensen referred to her hypothesis as "socioemotional selective theory".

achievement is that I did not become depressed. This is not surprising at all, as this agrees with the findings of Carstensen's research[64]. Carstensen's research demonstrated that as people become older, they become happier. They are less prone to anxiety, depression, and anger.

Despite this trend of increasing happiness, I am unsure how I will react when I can no longer make decisions on my own. Like the elderly people in retirement homes, there will be a point soon when I will be frail and probably have lost most of my cognitive abilities, where other people have to make decisions on my behalf.

2 October 2023: My Mum's burden

BBC headline: Alien life in Universe: Scientists say finding it is 'only a matter of time'

Today, I woke up very early. It felt like I had been awake most of the night. I am in the Netherlands, visiting my parents. I am staying in the same house where my grandparents lived most of their lives. My mind wandered whilst I was trying to remember the events that had occurred fifty years ago. Fifty years ago, I was lying in bed about 10 m away from the spot where I am currently lying. Back then, I also woke up early in the morning. I remember waking up whilst a ray of the morning sun shone across my bedroom onto the bed where I had spent the night underneath a heavy brown blanket. The blanket was "from the olden days" – it was unlike the lightweight duvets we had at home at that time. I was on holiday, "op vakantie", at my maternal grandparent's house. I used to lie in bed in deep concentration trying to make out the first noises that announced the start of a new day. After I was confident that the sounds were from my grandparents, I got up, went down the stairs, entered the kitchen, and sat down for my breakfast. Each morning, I saw my Grandma, who was normally busy in the kitchen. Most mornings, I saw my Granddad shuffling into the kitchen for his breakfast, only to shuffle to his chair and sit there for the rest of the day. I have a clear vision of Granddad sitting in his favourite chair whilst

---

[64] Recently, I was told a story about the wife of a colleague who became severely depressed when she searched the web and found the statistics of Overall Survival of the cancer she was suffering from. Carstensen's choice of words is very appropriate – "less prone to depression".

watching a football match on his black and white television. From a boy's perspective, his life seemed very boring.

Fifty years later, I listened to the sounds I could hear through the open window. I can hear the faint sound of the motorway – according to my Dad - the sound is like waves crashing on the beach in the far distance. I can hear the clicking sound of the clock hanging on the living room wall and the occasional car driving past the house. Dad was coughing in the adjacent bedroom. I heard his coughs throughout the night.

I spent the past 9 days at my parents. My sister-in-law had warned me about Dad's declining health. Initially, I did not recognise how much his health had declined, but over the following days, I changed my mind. Just like Granddad in the late 1970's, Dad shuffles behind his rollator from his bedroom bed to his bed standing in the living room. He has lost much of his strength in his legs, and his habitual walks and bike rides are no more than a fading memory.

Today, I am travelling back to the UK. I realise that I am leaving my parents in a very bad situation. A couple of days ago, I told my Dad that I will probably die before Spring. Spring 2024 is only 7 months away. I did not tell Mum. I simply could not face telling her. I fear that the news will push her beyond her breaking point. That same evening, I told my brother and sister-in-law. We planned how to inform my Mum. I fear that 2024 will be a horrible year for my Mum. I think that it is highly likely that once the end of 2024 is reached, Mum will have lost her husband, her son and her sister[65]....

While I am with my parents, they act as if everything is fine – as if there is no problem whatsoever. I believe this is normal behaviour for a caring parent – parents want to protect their children for as long as possible. I am as guilty of this behaviour as my parents are – you don't want to share the horrendous truth, the reality that we all die – eventually.

5 October 2023: What should I do after my book is finished?

BBC headline: Warmest September on record as 'gobsmacking' data shocks scientists

Over the past 18 months, I have spent much of my time writing my book. This book is now almost finished, and my expectation is that once the draft is accepted, I will fall into a hole. Twenty-three years ago, I fell into a similar hole

---

[65] My Mum's sister is suffering from pancreatic cancer.

after I submitted my Ph. D. thesis. The life crises that followed ultimately resulted in packing in my geology career. This time around, the result will be much more dramatic.

How should I use my time after I finish my book? What should I do with my spare time? What is next? I do realise the irony of the situation; I am mortally ill and I am talking about having too much time! I am very conscious of the fact that I am literally running out of time. Many months have been reduced to a few months. What should I do in these precious final months when I am healthy?

I feel a strong sense of guilt. Towards my children, I feel that I should have done more to support them. Towards my wife, I feel that I should have been a better husband. I do not want to be a burden on my family. Therefore, I decided to continue my normal working routine as long as I can physically do so.

A couple of months ago, I was contemplating writing another book. Along the lines of "don't make the same mistakes that I made 30 years ago." However, after a couple of days on the internet, I realised that there is already a massive amount of information freely available to advise young people[66]. No one is awaiting my kernel of wisdom. I also fear that there is simply not sufficient time left to bring the project to a successful conclusion.

I decided to write a letter to my children instead. At work, I decided to work on a series of short projects. The main aim is to transfer the knowledge I have acquired to the younger generation and ensure that they do not have to go through all the hard groundwork that I had to go through. I also have to finalise the book *Insight*. I suppose one could argue that I am trying to "build a legacy." I think the word "legacy" has a slightly negative meaning. It has a selfish ring. I just want to help the people around me…

20 October 2023: Failing to support my Dad and my Mum's sister

BBC Headline: Communities in Angus now only accessible by boat

Today, I realised that I failed to support my Dad and my Mum's sister. I should have done more to support my parents and my Mum's sister. Although I feel I should not be too harsh on myself, given the distance between us and the fact that there is only so much one can do during brief visits and over the phone.

---

[66] I believe that 80,000 hours is an excellent resource (https://80000hours.org/)

This week, Dad decided to reduce the pain medication he had been taking for the last year. The strength of the medication has increased dramatically. He used to take a relatively low dose of morphine, but over time he switched to fentanyl and methadone. I strongly suspect that his body is addicted to these opioids. I know that at this very moment, he is in great pain...Also, this week, my Mum's sister decided not to go ahead with another round of chemotherapy. She was really ill during her previous chemotherapy, so I understand her decision. I just hope she is not giving up.

I tried to define their value system by letting my parents and my Mum's sister put a set of cards in order of importance (I discuss the findings in the chapter Exploring different value systems). I hope that this exercise made my parents reflect on their value system and create some clarity about what is important to them. In my discussions with both my Dad and my Mum's sister, I applied the principles of Decision Quality. Although I did not mention Decision Quality by name, I went through all the decision elements to be sure that the decisions they were about to make were as good as they possibly could be.

Concluding remarks: Surviving

I hope that this description of my thinking process is useful to the reader. I tried using all the information that was available at the time when I was developing the decision models. I believe that one must be pragmatic when developing a decision model. I do realise that the way I structured the analysis is not perfect in any model. To me, that is a fact – a given. It is always possible to add more data from the internet or apply better logic, but the question is whether that effort would ultimately pay off. Would the decision be significantly better after you have gone through this effort? In the end, it is a personal choice how to construct your decision model. The insight created by a model is a function of the model itself. For example, the expected value of a decision tree will change when a couple of branches are added. This is expected. It is completely logical.

During my career, I spent years checking numbers and trying to find the reason why two models yielded different numbers. Typically, after weeks or months of work, I would realise that the observed difference could be explained by a rounding error or some other bit of logic that caused a slight difference in the calculated values. Was it worth the effort? Well, it did pay for the mortgage...

In the next chapter, I will reflect on my life and life in general.

Life

'...my wife (an oncologist I remind you) is in tears, every night and every time we discuss an event more than a year or so into the future. I think that says it all.

Adam Blain in *Pear Shaped*

'We need to stop feeling superior and special, seeing that death is a fate shared by us all. We are all a part of the brotherhood and sisterhood of death.'

Robert Greene in The Laws of Human Nature

'I should warn you that my head is bandaged because I have a brain tumour.'
– John Jr.
'I've never known anybody with a brain tumour.' – Boy
'You know me.' – John Jr.
'What's it like?' – Boy
'I've been lucky. I have no pain, and there has been no impairment of my faculties.' – John Jr.

John Gunther in *Death be not Proud*.

Abstract Life

Over the past 53 years, I have embraced living. I have lived life to the fullest. Live is a gift to every child, woman, and man alive. I have had many great experiences and met many fabulous people who have shaped me into the person that I am today.

I do realise that life can be a struggle at times. Grieving is one of those struggles. Someone close to you is suddenly gone – gone forever. To many of us, me being one of them, this realisation comes as a complete shock. In western culture, we do not know how to cope with death effectively. Dying is something that happens on the margins of our society – out of sight. We must become consciously aware that living and dying are intricately linked – there is no life without death.

Life-changing events that have shaped me

Recently, I reflected on the tragedies that my family has experienced over the years. My mum's youngest sister, Maria, was killed in a car crash aged 16. At the time, my Mum was expecting me, and after my birth, baby Bart was used as a weapon of distraction to my Grandma. I suspect that this resulted in a lifelong close connection between us. I have happy vacation memories of spending time with my Grandma; being sent to bed with two handfuls of sweets and waking up early in the morning listening to the first sounds in the house that signalled that I could get up. I don't think that my grandparents ever got over their loss. Many years later, after my Granddad had passed away, Grandma was still grieving for the daughter she had lost.

A second family tragedy occurred when the oldest cousin from my maternal side was killed. In 1991, Antwan, aged 20, was a second family victim of Dutch traffic. At the time, I was travelling in Spain with three university friends. Much later, I was told that my Grandma's initial thought was that it was me who was killed. Grandma was a very religious person and was informed by the local pastor. My uncle and aunt divorced soon after Antwan's death. Antwan's parents, like my Grandparents, never fully recovered from their loss.

My parents suffered from their fair share of health issues. My Dad fell ill with back problems in the early 1970s. After multiple failed attempts to relieve him from his back pains, he had to give up his profession as a road-building project manager. My Mum told me that Dad never opened the envelopes containing his final certificates. He hardly slept because of the pain, lost half his income overnight, and became severely depressed.

At the time, his doctor told him that by the time he would reach his mid-fifties, things might improve, and it did. By the time he reached early retirement, his pain had subsided. Ironically, a second boost to his health came after he was diagnosed with prostate cancer. After 30 odd years, he finally dropped his corset. This corset, a tight garment used to straighten his back, had been crushing his lungs for decades.

My Dad's passion was driving his motorhome. Since the 1970s, he and his father have owned over eight motorhomes. With his health issues sorted, Mum and Dad travelled throughout Europe and beyond: Nordkapp (northern point of Norway), Kurdistan (southern Turkey), South Africa, Morocco and Scotland!

In early 2020, whilst the COVID-19 pandemic triggered lockdowns in many parts of the world, my parents were in Morocco. They had to leave behind their beloved motorhome and were repatriated by the Dutch government. After landing at Schiphol airport, one of my cousins drove up from the southeast of the Netherlands to pick them up just after midnight. My sister-in-law had arranged for transport as they could not drive to the airport because my brother and his family were already experiencing COVID-19 symptoms.

The COVID-19 pandemic struck my parents hard. The two years of lock down were described by my Dad as "lost years"; years that were very precious to him.

Reflecting on my childhood, I now realise that my Dad was disabled for many years when my brother and I were growing up. Mum looked after us. In the 1970s–1980s, she worked as a dressmaker for her clientele. Somehow, in 1990, when Mum was in her early 50s, she befriended an old lady who had been in the embroidery business for a very long time. She borrowed my Mum an old sewing machine that enabled Mum to make large flags that are used by civic guards (*schutterijen*) in their annual processions. A few years later the elderly lady passed away and Mum took over the business. There was a reasonable amount of money to be made as each of the local villages had a civic guard, and all of them had local sponsors to pay for their costumes, weapons, and flags.

I do believe that a human being can only cope with a certain amount of cumulative stress and spend a finite amount of energy, and I somehow suspect that Mum's resources were drained by the mid-noughties. Gradually, she became increasingly anxious about ageing. She did not want to become frail.

In 1984, my parents moved into my mother's family home. The house was paid in cash by my granddad, my mum's Dad, for less than 2,000 guilders. In the 1940s, you could pick up some "prime property" for less than 1,000 British Pounds in a small village in the south-eastern part of the Netherlands – Brabant. While refurnishing the house, extra wide doors were fitted, and all rooms were on the ground floor. At this stage, my parents were expecting that my Dad would be confined to a wheelchair in a couple of years. A wheelchair was never wheeled in. That is, until very recently.

In the autumn of 2021, both my parents were rushed to the hospital in an ambulance. Dad was the first to be hospitalised. I vividly remember the long drive to the Netherlands from the UK not knowing in what state I would find my parents. My parents attempted to marginalise their problems, and my sister-in-law tried to correct the biased picture my parents painted. I left my parents a week later after Dad had returned home from the hospital. The following week, it was Mum who required hospital care. In the summer of 2023, Dad was bedridden again and was suffering from a lot of pain. Despite his failing health, Dad is still grateful for all the travels Dad and Mum took in their beloved motorhome, and he is still hoping for a full recovery.

My tumour does not qualify as a tragedy. The early deaths of Maria and Antwan prevented them from living their childhood dreams. Neither of them was able to execute their plans and ambitions and enjoy the full extent of their youth. Furthermore, I am completely free from pain. As a matter of fact, I have no discomfort whatsoever. I do not fear death, I am unafraid to die. I am happier today than I was before my tumour was found. However, my tumour will very likely prevent me from reaching old age. The prospect of frailty does not particularly appeal to me. In my early 50s, I am slowly but surely entering the final chapter of my life – old age.

I have been given the opportunity to make choices, have had an amazing set of life experiences, and have met many wonderful people. I have been in good health, unaffected by worries about money, for my entire adult life. I have met a wonderful wife, and I am truly blessed with our two children. I am grateful and happy for the life I had for the past 53 years.

WEIRD

WEIRD is a phenomenon that plagues psychology and other social science studies. Their participants are overwhelmingly Western and Educated and from Industrialised, Rich and Democratic countries. I am also WEIRD. Reflecting on this somewhat more, I am wEiRd: highly educated and (relatively) rich[67]. The statement "Money cannot buy happiness" is simply incorrect. If you do not have sufficient funds to feed your family, you will be very unhappy. Clearly, there is no linear relationship between the amount of money you have available and your happiness. The impact of 1,000 Euro on a poor person could be life changing. The same 1,000 Euro will have a much smaller impact on a very rich person – she might spend the money to buy a small jar of caviar. I am fortunate to having

---

[67] I never had any worries about a lack of money.

been continuously employed for the past 2 decades, which has allowed me to accumulate a decent nest egg. Even if I stopped working today, my wife and I have together accumulated a sum of money that is sufficient to keep us going for another four to five decades.

I realise that I am very fortunate. Recently, many people simply cannot make ends meet. The fact that the BBC has a section dedicated to the *cost of living*[68] highlights the extent of the problem. The BBC headline "1 in four working London parents struggle to feed their family" sums it up.

To me, being rich is also a proxy for having a high Quality of Life. A quarter of people in the UK are living with chronic pain. Those people clearly have a much lower Quality of Life than me (although this might well dramatically change in a couple of months…).

I am also highly educated. My university degrees include a *propedeuse* (a Dutch degree received upon completing the first year at university), a *doctoraal* (a Dutch degree received upon completing my geology degree, roughly equivalent to an MSc), a Ph.D. (a Danish degree from Copenhagen University), and finally an MBA (a Dutch degree from Nyenrode University). I found one online source[69] that claimed that in the Western world, only 1.1% of people hold a Ph.D. The combination of a Ph.D. and an MBA must, per definition, be rarer still. In addition, I have spent decades reading and writing academic manuscripts on a broad range of topics. During my life, I have collected a non-fiction library that consists of four sets of bookshelves.

The combination of having sufficient funds to take care of my family and the knowledge I have gathered over my life has pulled me through so far. I am personally convinced that my knowledge of statistics and decision sciences helped me to keep my thoughts straight and prevent me from worrying too much (although admittedly the tumour growing in my brain is constantly in the back of my mind. The tumour was actually located in the front!).

I recognise that people have different coping mechanisms. Religion is by far the most common coping mechanism, more than 90% of adults express a belief in God, and around 70% consider religion as one of the most important influences in their lives[70]. One of my Mum's aunts lit a massive candle for me, and she gave me a statue from the pilgrimage to Lourdes for moral support. One

---

[68] https://www.bbc.co.uk/news/topics/cljev4jz3pjt
[69] https://www.weforum.org/agenda/2019/10/doctoral-graduates-phd-tertiary-education/
[70] Gallup, 1996.

of my uncles led the prayers in the church to support me. Other coping mechanisms include seeking support from cancer support groups, mindfulness and relaxation (e.g., yoga), expressive arts (e.g., writing or painting). I am sure that many other options exist.

Some of us might choose to live in denial of their terminal disease. The latter option is not a coping mechanism, and I would not recommend this alternative.

The point is that "our griefs are as personal as our fingerprints".[71] My wEiRd approach, for the time being at least, works for me.

Grief

I might be at ease with my looming death, but I do have a family. I have a wife, two children, a brother, and parents who are all likely to experience a period of *grief*.

Grief was introduced to psychology by Freud's influential work on *Mourning and Melancholia*[72]. Grief is a strong, sometimes overwhelming emotion for people who have lost someone close to them. Those affected by grief find themselves feeling numb, lost, and unable to perform daily tasks. In her book *The Year of Magical Thinking*, Joan Didion writes: 'Grief comes in waves, paroxysms, sudden apprehensions that weaken the knees and blind the eyes and obliterate the dailiness of life' and 'The worst days will be the earliest days. We imagine that the moment to most severely test us will be the funeral…We anticipate needing to steel ourselves for the moment: will I be able to greet the people, will I be able to leave the scene, will I be able even to get dressed that day?…Nor can we know ahead of the fact (and here lies the heart of the difference between grief as we imagine it and grief as it is) the unending absence that follows, the void, the very opposite of meaning, the relentless succession of moments during which we will confront the experience of meaninglessness itself' and 'People in grief think a great deal about self-pity. We worry about it, dread it, scourge our thinking for signs of it. We fear that our actions will reveal the condition that is described as "dwelling on it." We understand the aversion that most of us have to "dwelling on it." Visible mourning of us of death, which

---

[71] Volkan and Zintl, 1993.

[72] Freud, 1917.

132

is construed as unnatural, a failure to manage the situation. Some people literally die of grief[73].

In his paper, *On Death and Dying,* Kübler-Ross[74] described a five-stage model of grief: shock and denial, anger, bargaining, depression, and acceptance. These stages can be recognised in both terminally ill patients and their family members. From personal experience, I can tell you that I have skipped a couple of these phases, and I have not been angry or depressed. I experienced a real shock when I was told that I had only 16 months to live (possibly because in my original survival model I estimated a 50% chance that I would get to 6 years). Jordan Peterson, in his book *12 Rules for Life* stated 'Life is in truth very hard. Everyone is destined for pain and slated for destruction.' I could not agree more with this point of view.

Over the summer of 2022, I read a Ph.D. thesis written by Elif Ünal[75] about *anticipatory grief.* Anticipatory grief has been defined as the presence of grief symptoms (e.g., longing/yearning for the person) while a family member with a terminal illness is still alive[76]. In contrast to popular belief, comparable levels of grief can be experienced in response to the expectation of loss as much as in the case of the loss itself[77].

Anticipatory grief was first introduced by Lindemann in 1944. Lindemann described anticipatory grief as a grieving process in anticipation of the death of a loved one. He proposed this, at the time, novel concept based on his observation that spouses of soldiers fighting in World War II rejected their returning husbands after the war. Lindemann assumed that these spouses had begun their grieving process and had detached their emotional bonds in anticipation of losing their husbands, who were unlikely to return from war. Anticipatory grief has been related to the families of terminally ill patients when a loved one's imminent death occurs rather than when a sudden death occurs[78].

During the anticipatory grief period, individuals tend to cope with the negative emotions provoked by a painful reality mostly by suppressing their

---

[73] Young et al., 1963; Rees and Lutkins, 1967

[74] Kubler-Ross, E., 1969.

[75] The majority of this chapter has been summarised from a thesis published in 2019.

[76] Lindemann, 1944; Nielsen et al., 2016.

[77] Ivancovich, 2004; Kehl, 2005; Rogalla, 2015.

[78] Fulton, 2003; Gerber et al.,1975; Sweeting & Gilhooly, 1990.

feelings[79]. They also prefer to distract themselves with caregiving duties or other daily tasks, rather than thinking about the possibility of death[80]. This tendency is rationalised as a necessity because being able to handle daily tasks or caregiving responsibilities requires that individuals not be overwhelmed by negative emotions[81]. Avoiding talking about death with family members, the sick person, or friends is another strategy individuals use in their attempt to cope with the proximity of death[82]. Another strategy for coping with anticipatory grief may involve detaching oneself from the dying loved one[83].

We are all turkeys

In *The Denial of Death*, Ernest Becker (1973) states that when children reach adulthood, they have learned that the length of their life is finite. Young adults have become aware of the fact that they are mortal. This realisation is a real shock to these young individuals. The transition that coincides with puberty from a fairy tale world of a child into an adult world that ends with a brutal miserable death is so shocking that most of us choose to ignore this reality. The author of the book *Four Thousand Weeks*, Oliver Burkeman[84], states, 'I don't live my own life in a permanent state of unflinching acceptance of my mortality.' Perhaps nobody does.' I believe most of us go through life avoiding the thought of death. Few of us are willing to engage in the thought of dying. I had been in denial of my own death until I fell ill. After a brain tumour was discovered inside my skull, I have been thinking about my own mortality every day.

The author of the book *The Laws of Human Nature*, Robert Greene[85], wrote, 'By becoming deeply aware of our mortality, we intensify our experience of every aspect of life.' I agree with the latter author when he writes, 'Understanding the shortness of life fills us with a sense of purpose and urgency to realise our goals' and 'We must think of our mortality as a kind of continual deadline. We must stop fooling ourselves: we could die tomorrow, and even if we live for another eighty years, it is just a drop in the ocean of the vastness of

---

[79] Clukey, 2008.

[80] Penrod et al., 2011.

[81] Sandilger & Cain, 2005.

[82] Spichiger, 2009.

[83] Ziberfein, 1999.

[84] Burkeman, 2021.

[85] Green, 2018.

time, and it always passes more quickly than we imagine. We must awaken to this reality.'

I remember a story about a turkey that Nassim Taleb told his YouTube audience. The story goes that it is entirely predictable that turkeys will be slaughtered before Christmas, but for the turkey, this is a complete shock. The turkey is fed every day for its entire life, so it looks forward to its daily meal. 1 day, the farmer shows up not with food but with an axe.

Recently, I have been thinking about turkeys a lot. Each morning after I get up, I visualise an image of a turkey. I shake my head to find out if I am in any pain. I know that I am one of these turkeys.

Whenever we enter a supermarket to buy a piece of turkey, we find the turkey meat nicely wrapped in a clinch film placed in a rectangular plastic tray. A label that states "turkey" enables the customer to distinguish turkey meat from chicken meat. Often, you will find a reference to the lower calorific value of turkey meat compared to chicken meat. I suspect that many people would not even recognise a living turkey. The gory process of butchering the poor turkey is best kept hidden from view. The process of chopping off the head from the turkey, skinning the animal, and removing its intestines is simply too much for the average shopping customer. The average shopper drops a rectangular plastic tray containing turkey meat into their shopping basket.

In our society, we deal with death similarly. We are obsessed by the young and beautiful and do not want to be confronted with the sick and dying. We stick the sick in hospitals and the elderly in care homes – out of sight. We check our phones for the latest pictures of a cute dog and focus on the latest film released by Netflix. Dying in contrast is something that takes place at the margins in our western culture. People die obscured from view – in private[86].

But remember, we are all turkeys waiting for the day that the axe will drop!

Concluding remarks: Life

Life is short. Even if we survive a couple more decades or even many more decades, our lives will still be short. You must make the most of this precious gift called "live" whilst being alive!

---

[86] In 1922, when Emily Post wrote her book Etiquette, the act of dying had not been professionalised. It did not typically involve hospitals. Woman died during childbirth. Children died of fever. Cancer is untreatable (Didion, 2005).

Part 3

Outline of part 3

The chapter *Communication* describes how to have an effective dialog and the requirements for such a dialog. Decision analysis is essentially a toolkit that supports communication – with others and with yourself. The following chapter, *Creativity*, provides a description of approaches to prevent tunnel vision. Although this topic is rarely discussed in the context of decision analysis, creativity is essential for becoming a better decision maker. *Values* stresses the importance of personal values, and in this chapter, the reader is introduced to the concept of objective networks. In the chapter *Decision analysis*, I take the reader through the process of decision analysis: framing, influence diagrams, decision trees, strategy tables, Multi-Criteria Decision Analysis and Decision Quality. In the next chapter, *Willingness to Pay*, I write about how people have tried to define a monetary amount that we as a society are willing to spend on the lives of human beings. In chapter *Innumeracy*, I discuss how both patients and doctors struggle with their understanding of statistics and what to do about it. In the chapter *Human judgement,* I introduce the techniques needed to develop high-quality judgements.

I used the colour coding of ski runs to mark the difficulty of the text: green, blue, red and black. The analogy is that a blue ski run might turn into a black run from the time it opens to the public with nice, compacted snow in the morning, changing to a mogul field with heavy sluggish snow in the afternoon. The ease of use of a certain technique depends on the decision at hand. For example, decision trees are easy to develop for some decisions, whereas for a slightly different decision, the decision tree will become unwieldy.

Communication

'How little do doctors understand the hells through which we put patients.'

Paul Kalanithi in *When Breath Becomes Air*

'In that first year, I would glimpse my share of death... At moments, the weight of it all became palpable. It was in the air, the stress and misery...I was in the hospital, trapped in an endless jungle summer, wet with sweat, the rain of tears of the families of the dying pouring down.'

Paul Kalanithi in *When Breath Becomes Air*

Abstract Communication

Decision analysis is all about effective communication. A dialogue that enables the patient and their family to express their wishes and discuss them with the medical team. I believe that over the recent years significant progress has been made and that hospitals are now more willing than ever before to engage with patients. However, it is the patient's role, their responsibility, to express their wishes. The principles discussed in this chapter should enable patients to express their wishes more effectively.

Another aspect of communication is to inform people who are close to you about your condition. One must be sensitive to those who are at the receiving end of the message; you are dropping a bombshell on them. Their lives will never be the same after you have spoken. Telling the people that are dearest to me the truth about what has just happened to me was the hardest thing I have ever done – ever.

The old science mantra – teach the public science and the public will understand complex science issues – has failed. One of the great paradoxes of today is that the public has greater access to high-quality scientific information than ever before. However, the offering of this knowledge is disrupted by overwhelming choices offered through a fragmented media system; hence, science enthusiasts become more knowledgeable, whereas the general audience literally tunes out. There is a need for innovative public engagement in research by designing messages that are personally relevant and meaningful to diverse publics, including patients.

Decision Hierarchy

[Difficulty: Green][87]

Decision analysis is not a single technique that can be applied to all problems. Instead, decision analysis should be considered a toolkit. You have a set of tools that can be applied to create insight, insights that trigger action.

I use decision hierarchy as an example of a decision analysis tool. Decision hierarchy is used to prioritise decisions by classifying each decision as a given, a decision for now, or a decision for later:

> Given (or fact): a decision that has been made or uncertainty that has been resolved;
> Decision for now: a decision that must be addressed now or;
> Decision for later: a decision that can be addressed at a later time.

As an example, imagine that you are planning to build a house. First, you submit bids for various plots of land. At this point, the location of your new house is a decision that is dependent on which bid for land results in a purchase. Once you have purchased a plot of land, the location of your house is no longer a decision; it has become a *given*.

Some decisions are simply irrelevant for now, such as the colour of the paint for the bedroom door, the pattern of the bathroom wallpaper or the material for the kitchen curtains. These decisions will become relevant in the future as you make the decision to proceed with the house build.

After your offer on the plot has been accepted, the immediate decisions will probably include whether to have a garage, whether to build a bungalow or a multi-storey building, and what the number of bedrooms should be.

---

[87] In this part of the book, I use ski run colour coding. Green is very easy, blue is easy, red is challenging, and black is very hard.

As the build progresses, also uncertainties are resolved. Initially, there might be uncertainties around planning permissions, but as the project progresses, these planning permissions will hopefully be granted. As you spend your budget, you get more clarity on the uncertainty around the funds remaining, and the uncertainty of what to do with this excess budget will get resolved. Each of these uncertainties will turn into a *given* the moment these uncertainties are resolved.

As each of these decisions gets resolved or an uncertainty is resolved, these issues will become a *given.* At this point, one or more decisions for later will become a *decision for now.*

Decision hierarchy is just one example of a tool that enables us to break down the complexity of a decision into smaller, more comprehensible parts. The commonality among all decision analysis tools is that they aid communication.

Effective dialog facilitated by decision analysis

[Difficulty: Green]

Decision analysis is a social activity. An effective dialogue is needed using simple language that, for example, can be used to explore trade-offs between options or to discuss uncertainties that have an impact on patient preferences. Such dialogue will enable the patient, their family, and their medical team to clearly articulate their wishes and beliefs regarding the options of a treatment plan and its implications for Quality of Life. The language of decision analysis will improve the articulation of options and uncertainties, which will translate into a richer dialog around decisions. The use of such language removes any ambiguity and makes the underlying concepts more precise and concrete. The introduction of a common language will ultimately enhance the stakeholders' commitment to follow through with the recommendations of the analysis.

Doctors practises voodoo and mysticism

[Difficulty: Green]

In the 1950s, the famous statistician Sir Ronald Aylmer Fisher wrote, 'A large number of the smokers of the world are not very clever, perhaps not strong minded. The [smoking] habit is insidious, difficult to break...'[88]. This statement, made by the inventor of the techniques that are used to this day when analysing data collected during clinical trials, denigrates the mental competence of many

---

[88] Gould, 1996.

lung cancer patients. Fifty years later, in 2000, Gerd Gigerenzer captured the following quotes at a medical conference: '60% of patients, conservatively estimated, do not have the intellectual capacity to make decisions about treatment themselves.' 'I tell women about cost and benefits so they can make up their minds. But few are interested in the numbers – most decide irrationally.' '[Patients] are anxious; they fear the worst; they want to be reassured.'

In March 2023, I attended a meeting with 10 doctors. The doctors were saying, 'patients are only interested in very basic facts, no details' and 'I am happy if they can pronounce the drug name.' But there were also other sounds in the room: 'patient is king', 'patients want the best care and are willing to suffer' and 'patient just want control of their life, a normal life without nausea, tiredness and depression. Patients want to spend time with their kids, travel, and have intimate relationships.

In May 2023, I asked David Spiegelhalter about changing attitudes towards patients. David told me that the curriculum of the training of doctors has evolved from a very much paternal role, which makes the decisions on behalf of the patient, to a much more patient-centric advisory role. Furthermore, David argued that particularly in rare diseases, patients are often more knowledgeable about their disease than the doctors who are treating them.

In July 2023, I interviewed a doctor who works at the cancer charity Maggies. Maggies and the NHS are cooperating where Maggies is providing psychological, emotional, and physical support and the NHS is providing medical, physical, and physical support. The doctor told me that she witnessed a change in attitude during her 30-year career. At present, there is an equal partnership between the doctors and patients, and on the various boards, there is always a patient present. This patient is empowered to ensure that changes can be made, e.g., changes regarding what data are collected or what services should be provided.

I believe that progress is being made. Recent conversations are very different from the gist of the two conversations that occurred over the past 70 years. To me, it seems we have finally turned a corner, we have empowered the patient.

There are other hopeful signs. Several special interest groups[89] have been established by patients, caregivers, and healthcare professionals. These special interest groups involve people who have come together around a common

---

[89] Special interest group in this context exclude groups that wish to exert political influence, as commonly seen in the United States.

interest and passion to share knowledge. Given that all their activities are online, group members do not have to be in the same location or even in the same country. These special interest groups extensively use podcasts, YouTube videos, and mailing lists. The concept of special interest groups was unknown before the widespread use of the internet.

In 2020, a recommendation was made to the NHS to develop a training programme for clinicians to have conversations with patients, particularly those who are at risk of dying in the next 12 months[90]. The aim of the conversations between health care professionals and patients is to provide patients with information about their condition and treatment options and to give them the opportunity to have their values, goals, priorities, and treatment preferences heard and respected by clinical staff.

Healthcare administrators recognise that clinicians have often not been sufficiently trained to feel comfortable initiating these conversations. However, these discussions are fundamental to effective clinical management plans. Given the increasing proportion of people living with one or more long-term conditions, it is more important than ever that we do not shy away from these conversations.

There is strong evidence that advance care planning and a subsequent earlier transition to palliative care can improve patients' satisfaction with the care they receive[91]. An earlier transition to palliative care has also been demonstrated to improve family satisfaction and reduce stress, anxiety, and depression in surviving relatives[92].

A culture of meeting performance targets and pressure within the health care system does not always permit physicians and other clinicians to prioritise proactive conversations in a clinic or on the ward. However, there might be more fundamental issues.

Medical staff should be fully aware of the asymmetry of their relationship with patients. Medical staff are experts, and patients are laypersons. In contemporary society, doctors and scientists are experts in that they hold a body of dominant knowledge that is, overall, inaccessible to the layman[93]. However, this inaccessibility and perhaps even the mystique that surrounds expertise does

[90] https://www.england.nhs.uk/wp-content/uploads/2021/07/SQW-NHS-England-Improving-communications-report-30June.pdf
[91] Gade et al., 2008; Detering et al., 2010.
[92] Orford et al., 2019.
[93] Fuller, 2005.

not cause the layman to disregard the opinion of the experts because of the unknown. Instead, the complete opposite occurs, whereby members of the public believe in and highly value the opinion of medical professionals or scientific discoveries despite not understanding them[94].

Consider carefully how you frame your expertise

Historically, a prevailing assumption has been that ignorance is the root of the lack of interest in science[95]. As a solution, after formal education ends, popular science media should be used to educate the public. Once citizens are brought up to speed on science, they will be more likely to judge scientific issues as scientists do, and controversy will disappear. In this traditional "popular science" model, communication is defined as a process of transmission. The facts are assumed to speak for themselves and to be interpreted by all citizens in similar ways. If the public does not accept or recognise these facts, the failure in the transmission is blamed on journalists, "irrational" beliefs, or both[96].

The great paradox of today's media world is that by way of cable TV and the Internet, the wider public has greater access to quality information about science than at any time in history, yet public knowledge of science remains low. One major reason is the problem of choice: citizens not only select media content based on ideology or religious views but also on their preference, or lack thereof, for public affairs and science-related information[97]. As a result, in a fragmented media system, information-rich science enthusiasts become richer, whereas the broader American audience literally tunes out[98].

Nisbet[99] argued that there is nothing essentially unique about science policy debates. Doctors must strategically *frame* their communications in a manner that connects them with their patients. Nisbet identified a consistent set of frames that appear repeatedly in science policy debates and then explained how this research might be turned into an innovative public engagement. This means that the science must be translated into messages that are personally relevant and meaningful to the diverse public, including patients.

---

[94] Fuller, 2005.

[95] Nisbet, 2009.

[96] Nisbet and Goidel, 2007.

[97] Prior, 2006.

[98] Nisbet, 2009.

[99] Nisbet, 2009.

Talking to medical doctors

[Difficulty: Green]

Although I have been treated very well by my medical team, I do feel that serious risks are embedded in the current medical system. I feel this is relevant because I suspect that many patients lack the ability to make the right treatment choices.

The public relies on the heuristic: 'If you see a white coat, trust it.' However, can you really rely on this rule of thumb? I would argue that doctors wearing "these white coats" are faced with a conflict of interest. Much of their continuing education is given in events sponsored by the pharmaceutical industry[100]. Doctors also have an incentive to overtreat (treatment for a medical condition that you would not have noticed in your remaining life span) and overdiagnoses (illnesses that have no impact on your remaining life span) because doctors, certainly in the USA, have a fear of potential lawsuits for negligence.

There are these protocols that follow. Protocols are a recipe for treating patients. For example, my treatment consisted of the following sequence of steps: 1) removal of the brain tumour, 2) 1-month recovery, 3) six weeks of chemo and radiation treatment, 4) 1-month recovery, 5) six months of chemotherapy, and 6) one scan every three months. If not for a recurrence of cancer growth that was detected during one of these routine 3 monthly scans, the three-monthly scans would have continued for a couple of years, followed by two scans a year for a couple of years and then an annual scan until recurrence, at which point further protocols come in, or non-brain tumour-related death. The objection I have with these protocols is that doctors could follow them blindly, failing to consider that the optimal treatment plan for an individual patient may well be different from the standard treatment protocol.

There is a simple solution to this conundrum by simply asking the treating physician: 'If I were your Dad/Mum, what would your advice be?'

Fisher's error

[Difficulty: Green]

Few readers have probably heard of Sir Ronald Aylmer Fisher (1890–1962). He did not write for the general public; he wrote about statistics. His pages and pages of mathematical formulae would be impenetrable to the layman and even

---

[100] Angel, 2004.

challenging to scientists. Even naturalists who study natural history are put off by his writing, even though his book *The Genetical Theory of Natural Selection* is a major contribution to what has been labelled "modern evolutionary theory". However, among statisticians, Fisher is a true hero.

Fisher, however, made a big mistake. Fisher was a smoker, and at the end of his career, he spent a considerable amount of effort trying to debunk the idea that smoking can cause lung cancer. There was a strong correlation between smoking and lung cancer[101], but that did not prove that smoking was the cause of lung cancer.

Fisher wrote in 1958, 'The pre-cancerous condition involves a certain amount of slight chronic inflammation. A slight cause of irritation is commonly accompanied by pulling out a cigarette and receiving a little compensation for life's minor ills. To take the poor chap's cigarettes away from him would be rather like taking way his white stick from a blind man[102].

Since Fisher wrote these lines, the medical community has gathered overwhelming evidence that smoking cigarettes is the single biggest risk factor for lung cancer. It is responsible for more than 7 of 10 cases of cancer. Tobacco smoke contains more than 60 known carcinogens (cancer producers). If you smoke more than 25 cigarettes a day, you are 25 times more likely to develop lung cancer than someone who does not smoke[103]. In 2020, 2.21 million cases of lung cancer were diagnosed worldwide[104].

Cancer arises from the transformation of normal cells into tumour cells in a multi-stage process that generally progresses from a pre-cancerous lesion to a malignant tumour. These changes result from the interaction between a person's genetic factors and three categories of external agents:

1. Physical carcinogens, such as ultraviolet (UV) and ionising radiation;
2. Chemical carcinogens, such as asbestos, tobacco smoke components, alcohol, aflatoxin (a food contaminant), and arsenic (a drinking water contaminant); and

---

[101] Correlation is the tendency of two variables to move in tandem, i.e., if one variable increases its value, so does the other variable (which is called a positive correlation).
[102] Gould, 1996.
[103] https://www.nhs.uk/conditions/lung-cancer/causes/
[104] https://www.who.int/news-room/fact-sheets/detail/cancer

3. Biological carcinogens, such as infections caused by certain viruses, bacteria, or parasites.

The incidence of cancer dramatically increases with age, most likely due to a build-up of risks for specific cancers that increase with age. The overall risk accumulation is combined with the tendency for cellular repair mechanisms to become less effective as a person grows older. Tobacco use, alcohol consumption, unhealthy diet, physical inactivity, and air pollution are risk factors for cancer[105].

Inform your family, friends, and colleagues

[Difficulty: Green]

Let me be very clear – there is no single optimal way to tell the people you care about most about your illness. Different people have different considerations that translate into highly personalised approaches. Because each person is unique, each of us has a specific way of dealing with the difficult issue of breaking the news about their illness. For example, I have two friends who are both cancer patients and are hesitant to share the news about their illness with a broad number of people. For very different reasons. One friend simply does not want people to know that he has cancer. The second friend is afraid that by sharing this knowledge, his career prospects will be affected. Recently, an aunt of mine was diagnosed with cancer, and she asked her son to reach out to her family on her behalf. She could not face the challenge of telling the news in person.

However, if you will tell people about your illness, there are some general rules that I feel apply in general. It has to do with communication. Your communication must be tailored to the person or audience you are talking to. With some people, you might choose a direct honest dialog, but to other people, one should be very sensitive about how to break the news. The words you choose, the pace of the conversation, and the length of time you pause between two sentences. One must be sensitive to those who are at the receiving end of the message; you are dropping a bombshell on them. Their lives will never be the same after you have spoken.

---

[105] https://www.who.int/news-room/fact-sheets/detail/cancer

I believe that there are three relevant dimensions in the communication process:

The degree the news affects the receiver;
The amount of information shared;
Perceived emotional fragility.

Figure 4.1 and 4.2 show my judgement on how the news of my disease impacted the receiver.

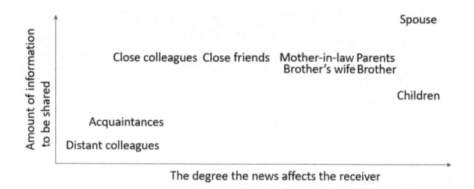

Figure 4.1. The amount of information shared and the degree to which the news affects the receiver.

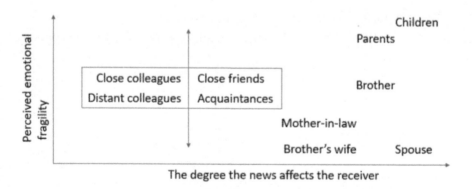

Figure 4.2. Perceived emotional fragility and the degree the news affects the receiver.

In my case, the people most affected by my terminal illness are my spouse and our children. My illness is likely to be fatal; therefore, there is no long-term future for me. Once I die, my wife becomes a widow and my children no longer have their father. My parents are also strongly affected. Most parents believe that they will be outlived by their children, and it must have been a real shock to them to be told that that is not going to happen because of my illness. My brother will lose his only sibling, and he will be forced to face the future without my wise words[106]. Close friends are affected, more so than close colleagues and acquaintances.

How much you tell these different stakeholders is a decision you will have to make. I made a choice to be completely open to people I knew reasonably well. I choose not to tell colleagues that I do not know well. Where you draw that line – who will you tell and who you won't – is a very personal choice.

I would also recommend setting a date for when you will inform people. Setting a date will enable you to plan the conversations that you will have and bring closure to this very difficult time.

In the chapter *Surviving,* I added more details on these very difficult but necessary conversations.

Concluding remarks: Communication

Communication is very important. Communication creates a common understanding of the situation. Communication ensures that we have all the facts and an awareness of the options and uncertainties.

The next topic is creativity. Communication and creativity are closely related. As Tim Brown from IDEO once stated, 'asking a question is a creative act.'

---

[106] I hope that my advice was somewhat useful.

Creativity

'...cancer forces deep reflection, causing you to think about the purpose and meaning of your life.'

David and Tom Kelley in *Creative Confidence*

Abstract Creativity

Creativity is essential when defining your value system, your decisions, the choices for the decisions, and the consequences of those choices in your decisions. Creativity broadens the mind and is essential as an antidote to tunnel vision. A lack of creativity is often the main reason why people struggle to create a comprehensive list of truly distinct perspectives.

The creativity of children is greatly diminished while they are growing up. By the time adults reach the age of 30, they are typically embarrassed to be involved in creative activities. Various techniques are described that stimulate creative thinking, and advice is given if you want to become more creative.

In contrast to children's creativity, which seems to take no effort at all, being creative as an adult can be challenging. Creativity demands cognitive resources, and creative sessions are generally accompanied by a sense of unnerving uncertainty and anxiety. However, creativity can also be fulfilling, purposeful, playful, and satisfying to our natural curiosity.

Creativity is also a choice – one must make a conscious choice to become creative

A deflating creative experience

[Difficulty: Green]

In 1981, aged eleven, I walked up to the front of my classroom to see my teacher, Mr. Van Dalen[107], who was grading the drawings made by my fellow pupils from my class. I was very proud of the drawing I had made. It was a drawing of a ship that was entirely in black and white. I used a single pencil, and by varying the pressure I applied to the pencil, I created different shades of grey. This created an effect that I found to be very effective. I believed that this drawing was fundamentally different from the artwork that my fellow class members produced at the time. A typical drawing of a ship produced by my fellow class members consisted of a blue wavy line for the sea at the bottom of the drawing, a basic outline of a boat drawn in brown, a few stick-like figures on the boat representing the captain and its crew, and a yellow sun in the top corner with rays of light emitting from it. These drawings were typically created using bright coloured felt-tip pens.

I remember getting in line behind two of my classmates who had produced two versions of a drawing in the felt-tip-pen-style. The first boy got his grade, and the second boy got a higher grade than the first boy. Now it was my turn. I remember putting my drawing on the desk of Mr. Van Dalen. He took a quick glance at the picture and scribbled a grade on my precious drawing. Mr. Van Dalen had given me the lowest of the three grades; in his view, my drawing was the least impressive of the three drawings he had graded. I vividly remember walking back to my desk feeling numb and deflated. I felt I had failed.

Two years later, I started at a new school. In the first week, I made a drawing that was hailed by the teacher as an example for all pupils to aspire to. That evening, I struggled to fall asleep from sheer excitement!

The fact that I have a very clear recollection of these two rather "mundane" events four decades later is a clear demonstration of the lasting impact these episodes had on me. Over the years, I have shared this story many times. On several of those occasions, people shared their own version of a similar creative-deflating event that had affected them.

It takes a lot of creative confidence to recover from these experiences.

---

[107] I suddenly realised that I do not actually know the given name of Van Dalen. He was always addressed as "Mr. Van Dalen" by the children.

Declining creativity when growing up

[Difficulty: Green]

A few years ago, I gave a series of presentations on the topic of creativity. After introducing the general topic, I asked the audience to draw the person sitting next to them. After I had asked the question, typically the room fell silent, followed by some voices making excuses – 'sorry, but I have not drawn in decades'; 'I am not an artist'; or 'I can't draw.' I was always amazed by this sense of awkwardness and unease. The audience was deeply embarrassed when asked to make a simple drawing. I never repeated this experiment with a room full of children, but I am convinced that the reaction would be very different. Children simply grab a pencil and with a few lines, create a drawing of their mama and papa (Figure 5.1).

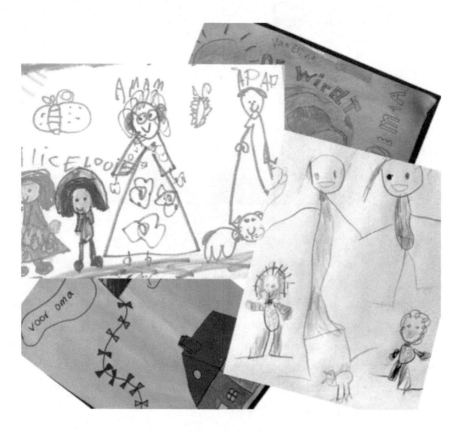

Figure 5.1. Children's drawings.

George Land designed a creativity test while working at NASA to screen for creative minds among their job applicants. Later, Land executed a research programme using the test he developed on 1,600 five-year-olds. The test indicated that 98 % of the children scored in the "highly creative" range (Figure 5.2). A second study discovered that children of similar age are the most curious, asking an incredible 390 questions every single day[108]. When Land re-tested these same children five years later, only 30 % of these 10-year-olds were still rated "highly creative". By the age of 15, only 12% of them were ranked in this category. A mere 2 % of 280,000 adults over the age of 25 years who had taken the same tests were still on this level. 'What we have concluded,' wrote Land, 'is that non-creative behaviour is learned.'

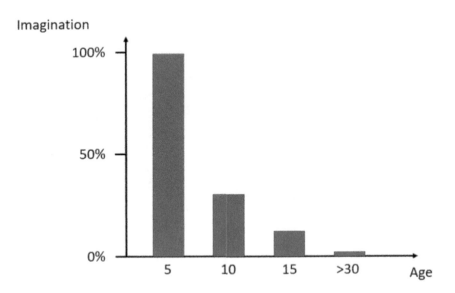

Figure 5.2. George Land's Creativity Test Results

The reason children are so creative is that they look at the world with fresh eyes[109]. When young children first come to school, everything is new and exciting. The world is awaiting them. They have an overwhelming need to explore life, have fun, and learn at the same time alongside their peers. They are always collecting information, data, and particulars that they eventually compile together. Everything is a new experience.

---

[108]https://www.timeslive.co.za/sunday-times/lifestyle/2013-03-31-kids-ask-390-questions-a-day/
[109] Shapiro, 2001.

154

However, once they start going to school and socialising with other children, they are forced to fit in. Peer pressure drives conformity. Education focuses on the regurgitation of facts rather than on gathering new experiences. Within a school and at university, students specialise and become proficient in a narrow, specific area. Once we enter the corporate world, staff are stigmatised for their mistakes. Corporate employees cannot have original, creative ideas if their environment does not allow them to fail. Our creative side is actively discouraged from blossoming. We can conclude that creativity is therefore not learned but rather unlearned[110]. However, creative abilities can be regained swiftly – even decades later.

Mindset

[Difficulty: Green]

People with a growth mindset believe that a person's true potential can be improved by training, passion, and toil. Carol Dweck, in her book *Mindset*, makes the case that people with a growth mindset can self-improve regardless of their initial talent, aptitude, or even intelligence. On the other hand, people with a fixed mindset have a fundamental belief that individuals are born with a certain amount of talent and intelligence. Individuals with a fixed mindset prefer to stay in their comfort zone and are afraid that their limitations will be exposed. In contrast, people with a growth mindset are much more willing to venture into creative activities and reach out into the unknown.

Growth mindset

To create an environment of fresh thinking, to inspire and generate ideation, a mindset of continuous innovation is essential. Fresh thinking and high levels of creative behaviour will enrich individuals' skills in critical thinking, problem solving and decision making. We want to fuse the curiosity and excitement we had towards the world as children, when almost everything seemed enchanted, with our adult intelligence[111]. The recreation, reliving, and childhood combined with the experience of an adult make a very powerful combination.

Creativity is not a brilliant idea that pops out of nowhere, but it is about looking at the world differently. Creativity is about listening and asking

---

[110] Shapiro, 2001.

[111] Greene, 2018.

unexpected questions that lead to unexpected answers[112]. To ask the right questions, one needs knowledge. Hence, knowledge is a key requirement for creative thinking. Breakthrough thinking is often the result of making novel connections a fresh approach to re-using concepts innovatively. Looking at a problem from a novel perspective can lead to the creation of novel associations and find analogies and metaphors.

Creativity allows one to see the world more clearly, unclouded by anxiety and doubt. Creativity is about believing in your ability to create changes in the world around you. This self-assurance, this belief in your creative capacity, lies at the heart of innovation.

You must make a choice to be creative. After you make this choice, you must persevere, accept failure, and have some fun during the journey. Perseverance is important because some of the best ideas originate from some of the most unlikely combinations and abstract references. The longer the list of ideas, the higher the quality of the final solution. Quite often, the highest quality ideas appear at the end of the list.

Fixed mindset

Childhood is a time of great emotional intensity. Once we become adults, this intensity diminishes, and gradually, we become more concerned with how others perceive us.

Because of this increased self-awareness, adults are afraid to ask "dumb questions" – particular questions that one "ought to know the answer to". In addition, many adults stop evolving and become locked into certain habits, ideas, and values[113]:

> Read the same sections of the newspaper;
> Watch the same style of movies;
> Narrow down the variety of foods they eat and;
> Socialise with the same friends.

---

[112] Brown, 2023.
[113] Shapiro, 2001.

Adults tend to find ways of functioning within our lives that work for us. Over time, instead of broadening their minds, adults continue to diminish their curiosity and creativity.

Knowledge is, in many ways, the enemy of creativity[114]. Once the human brain finds a satisfactory solution, it stops searching for alternatives. Unfortunately, these solutions may not be innovative or even good.

Design thinking

[Difficulty: Blue]

Being creative is hard work. On one hand, it is crucial to maintain momentum, while at the same time, it is important to have frequent breaks. Design thinking is a process that can accommodate a series of iterations or cycles that ensure that you are progressing but also that forces the person to take regular breaks to reflect. In software development, Agile is a common approach that aims to break down the workflow into a short burst of activity, followed by user testing, feedback collection, and a period of reflection[115].

A similar approach can be used for creativity (Figure 5.3):

1. Saturation: Absorbing knowledge. Interact with experts, read widely, deeply, and empathise. Followed by sorting, evaluating, organising outlining, and prioritising.
2. Incubation: Incubation involves mulling over information, "sense making" and recognising patterns. Walking away from the problem.
3. Illumination: Much of the maturation of ideas occurs subconsciously. Exploration of new possibilities and "ah-ha" moments.
4. Capturing ideas: Create a list of ideas by, for example, drawing a Mind Map (see section below).

---

[114] Although knowledge is also a requirement for creativity. See the section *Growth mindset*.

[115] In the Agile framework, which is applied to software development, these bursts of activity are referred to as Sprints, and the Minimal Viable Product is the software product that is tested by the users.

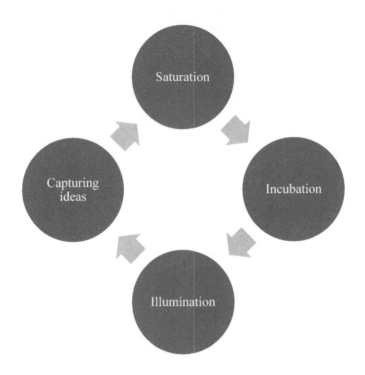

Figure 5.3. Cycle of saturation, incubation, illumination, and capturing ideas.

Kelley and Kelley, in their book *Creative Confidence*, state: 'Design thinking relies on the natural – and coachable – human ability to be intuitive, to recognise patterns and to construct ideas that are emotionally meaningful as well as functional' and 'We're not advising…to run an organisation solely on feeling, intuition and inspiration. But an overreliance on the rational and the analytical can be just as risky.'

Mind Mapping

[Difficulty: Blue]

Mind Maps can be used to capture all the ideas raised during a brainstorming session. Mind Mapping stimulates creative thought as you connect concepts and apply associative, diverging, and creative thinking. Mind Maps should be used early in the creative process to develop ideas.

The use of Mind Maps is an intuitive and structured way to capture and organise your thoughts. Mind Maps helps to clarify your thinking.

Mind Maps are useful for:

Brainstorming (individually or in groups);
Stimulating your creativity;
Research and consolidate information from multiple sources;
Gaining insight into complex subjects (patterns);
Studying and memorising information;
Communication ideas;
Problem solving;
Taking notes and;
Planning.

Drawing a Mind Map

Unlike other visual diagrams, a mind map is built around a single central topic[116]. This central topic is placed in the centre of a blank page. From the central topic, tree-like branches form the Mind Map (Figure 5.4). As you incorporate more ideas into the Mind Map, the diagram branches into topics and subtopics. The hierarchy of information that emerges is defined by the creator through categorizations and connections.

The structure of a Mind Map enables you to categorise and subcategorise information. Categorization helps our brains make sense of complexity. Mind Maps provide a hierarchical category structure that helps us navigate information more easily.

There is a temptation to use sentences in a Mind Map. However, it is very important to use single keywords. Another point that should be stressed is that the human mind struggles with holding too much information at once[117]. So, no more than 7 branches can originate from a single point in the Mind Map. Simplification is key!

---

[116] For more details, visit: https://www.mindmaps.com/what-is-mind-mapping/
[117] Psychological research has demonstrated that humans struggle to keep more than five or seven ideas in their brain at once.

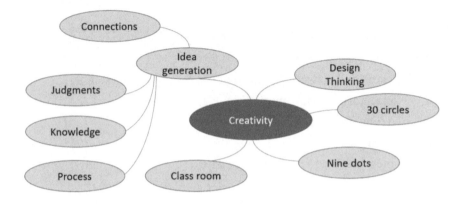

Figure 5.4. An example of a Mind Map.

Approaches for stimulating creative thoughts

[Difficulty: Green]

Active listening

Questions should inspire, fuel passion, provoke strong emotions, spur people into action, and lead to profound insights. Good questions relate to what you could do, not what you should do. Good questions trigger actions and create a proactive mindset.

Active listening requires commitment to be absolutely and totally in the conversation. The person should be curious, patient, and willing to be quiet to prevent the interruption of the person's thoughts. I recommend asking follow-up questions. In particular, if something is unclear and to playback to ensure you have fully understood the person you are engaging with.

Bob McKim Thirty circles

A simple creativity test is the thirty circles test proposed by Bob McKim (Figure 5.5). The objective of this test is to make as many drawings as possible using the thirty circles.

30 CIRCLES TEST

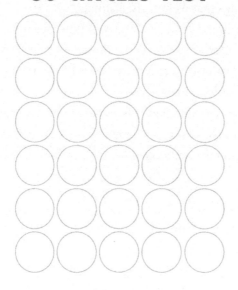

Figure 5.5. Bob McKim's thirty circles test.

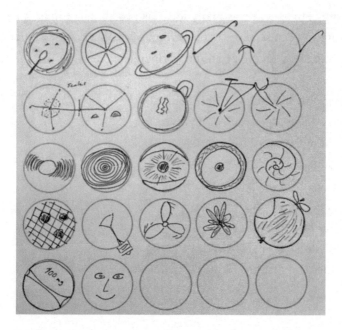

Figure 5.6. My personal results from the thirty circles test.

When I was generating my drawings, I was balancing two objectives: fluency (the speed and quantity of ideas) and flexibility (ideas that are truly different and distinct). I spent a couple of minutes whilst creating Figure 5.6, and I tried to come up with drawings that were truly distinct. I also tried to complete as many drawings as possible in the shortest amount of time. Admittedly, some drawings are a bit difficult to interpret, such as the drawing on the left in the second row from the top. This is a drawing of scales viewed from the top down. Well done if you interpreted this picture correctly!

We know from experience that it is easier to have a great idea if you have many to choose from. However, if you have many ideas that are just variations on a theme, you might have only one idea with twenty-nine other versions.

Brainstorming

Alex F. Osborn, the inventor of brainstorming, stated, 'brainstorming means using the brain to storm a creative problem and to do so in commando fashion, with each stormer audaciously attacking the same objective.'[118]

Over the past 6 decades, brainstorming has become a well-known approach to creating a list of ideas in a creative, unstructured manner. While brainstorming, an initial idea is used to stimulate other ideas (piggybacking). The objective of brainstorming is to generate as many ideas as possible in a short time.

Brainstorming can be done with a group of people or by a single individual. However, there are a couple of guiding principles:

> The problem should be well defined;
> Involve everyone – celebrate diversity;
> Encourage cross-fertilisation;
> Encourage outside-the-box thinking;
> Don't overlook the obvious;
> Suspend judgement;
> Do not fear repetitions;
> Don't stop and discuss and;
> Capture and display all ideas.

---

[118] Osborn, 1963.

Stay positive

When adults discuss a project, they tend to be sceptical and judgemental: 'We already tried that,' 'That is not practical,' 'That is a bad idea,' or 'This will never work.' In addition to the negativity, adults frequently pass judgement and do not add to the discussion of the ideas presented.

Positive: One must be positive in one's communication.

Have fun, use humour, and build on ideas that others have suggested. Ask questions like 'What could make it better?', 'What if...?', 'Could you just explain...?' or a simple ask 'Why?[119]'

Coe Leta Stafford brings to life the questions she is asking. So instead of asking 'Why do you like this book so much?', she will ask 'Pretend you wanted to convince a friend that they should read this book, what would you tell them?' By reframing the question, a game is created that yields much more insightful and meaningful answers.[120]

When asking these questions, a creative spark will ignite, and people will engage with your intellectual curiosity, deep optimism, and be more forgiven in your failures – I guarantee you that you will fail – repeatedly.

Importance of a process

Being creative is a choice. You should choose to be creative. Once you have made that choice, it is vital that the creative process does not lose momentum. We must ensure that the process continues to move forward. This is rather straightforward to achieve in a business context where you gather all stakeholders in a room or in a conference call for a pre-specified time window. Before the meeting, you can prepare an agenda specifying a list of topics and the time that the stakeholders can spend discussing each topic. In the case of a terminal illness, there will be meetings in the patient's diary that will provide natural deadlines. These deadlines provide guardrails for arranging goals that must be achieved within a certain time frame.

I recommend meeting in a quiet space where people can relax, be playful, ponder, and be curious. There should be a central topic around which all thoughts can evolve. I would advise that the session should be long enough so that participants can deal with trivial thoughts that people have to deal with, such as

---

[119] It is actually advisable to repeat the "why"-question four or five times.
[120] Kelley and Kelley, 2014.

arranging another meeting, making a phone call, buying a gift for their partner, and contemplating what needs to be done for a looming deadline. Ninety or hundred 20 minutes should be long enough to enter the creative zone and to get some creative thoughts. Many of the best ideas will come towards the end of the session when people have sufficient pondering time.

People will become bored during the session. The most creative people are those who are able to resist the temptation to decide and are more willing to continue despite this feeling of unease, this unnerving uncertainty. Creative people do not rush to judgements; instead, they are willing to "go-wide" first, identifying a number of possible approaches before converging on a single idea that is most worth implementing[121].

John Cleese describes the notion of open and closed modes[122]. Closed modes are good for decision-making and processes, whereas open modes are required to be creative. John stresses the need for both modes to be used and suggests that humour is an effective way to switch from one mode to the other. I once attended a meeting of fellow brain tumour patients, their partners, and carers. Although we discussed cancer and death, the lasting memory of that meeting was that there was a lot of laughter – people might be unlucky to end up with a terminal illness – but this does not prevent them from having a laugh!

Creating a creative list of ideas

[Difficulty: Green]

Creativity is a key factor in being successful in life. In 2010, IBM interviewed 1,500 CEOs across 60 countries. IBM concluded that 'Creativity is the most essential skill for corporations to succeed in an increasingly complex world' and 'To succeed…find new ideas and keep innovating in how to lead and communicate.' In my opinion, creativity is one of our most precious resources. It can help us find innovative solutions to some of our most intractable problems.

Peter Gray argued that 'you cannot teach creativity, you can only blossom it'[123]. Kelley and Kelley stated in their book *Creative Confidence*, 'Creativity is

---

[121] Kelley and Kelly, 2014.

[122] https://www.youtube.com/watch?v=Pb5oIIPO62g

[123] Gray, 2013.

like a muscle – it can be strengthened and nurtured through effort and experience.' John Cleese argued that creativity is a "way of operating"[124].

It is difficult to be creative when being put on the spot. This is illustrated by story Ralph Keeney told me about a group of doctoral engineering students at MIT. Ralph asked the students to write down a list of their personal objectives. Most of them wrote down a single answer. After some encouragement, the students added one or two more. Ralph told me that he had a list of more than 20 objectives. I recognise the difficulties these students faced. It is very hard to find a comprehensive list of items that capture one's complete value system. Likewise, it had to define a list of all decisions, choices for each decision, and the consequences of each of these choices. Once you start listing ideas, set yourself a high target. Try to get to 25 ideas. Persevere and do not give up!

The ideas described in this chapter are shown in Figure 5.7. The figure schematically illustrates how the ideas can be linked together to create a sufficiently long list of ideas.

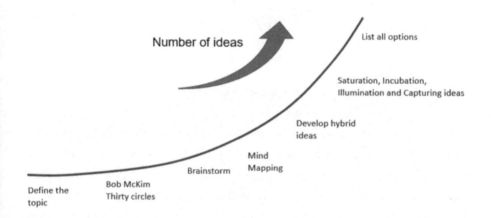

Figure 5.7. Creative process of developing ideas

Creativity over generations

[Difficulty: Green]

My favourite toy as a boy was Lego®. I have spent many years building Lego® models. I created planes, houses, spacecraft, cars, trains, bulldozers, and cranes. To me, even a wheel as pictured in Figure 5.8 was not just a wheel. I

---

[124] https://www.youtube.com/watch?v=Pb5oIIPO62g

transformed these wheels into windmills, Mississippi-style paddle boats, helicopters, cogs, and railroad carriages by sticking Lego® plates to the wheels or by running an elastic band over them (after removal of the rubber tyre). I would keep building until I ran out of bricks.

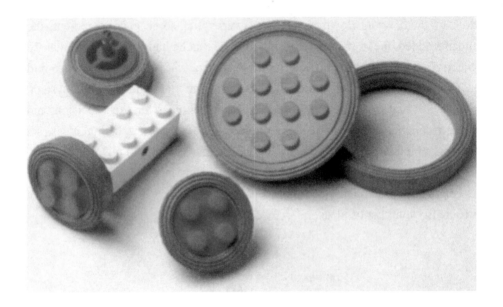

Figure 5.8. Lego wheels in the 1970s.

Thirty years later, I would buy Lego® sets for our son. Over time, many more different types of bricks were introduced by Lego. Soon, we found ourselves submerged in literally thousands of different Lego pieces[125]. My wife and I spend hours sorting all these bricks using different systems – by colour or by functionality – using one of these purpose-built systems with many drawers. This was a far cry from my childhood memories. This was sheer boredom! Instead of being creative, we spend our time sorting Lego®.

While my wife and I were sorting these gigantic piles of Lego®, our son discovered Minecraft®. In Minecraft®, you create a virtual world in which you build stuff. It is like virtual Lego®. Our son played Minecraft® for many years. He did not mind that the figures that appeared in Minecraft® had square heads,

---

[125] Moreau and Engeset (2016) argued that over the years, Lego has shifted its focus to kits that build single models as opposed to kits that can be reassembled into many models. This shift involved the need for many new bricks with few general applications.

nor did he mind that the way these figures moved around on his screen was somewhat jerky. He did play other games as well – he went through his Fortnite-phase – but he always returned to Minecraft®. Our son was playing Minecraft® the same way I used to play with Lego®. Submerged in creativity!

In the end, we sold off all the Lego® – including the Lego® bricks I used to play with in the late 1970s – and our son made a few hundred pounds in profit. All that remains is some beloved memories of my creative endeavours.

Out-of-the-box thinking: Nine-dot problem

[Difficulty: Red]

The task of the nine-dot problem: 'Can you draw four straight lines that connect all nine dots without lifting the pencil from the paper, see Figure 5.9?'

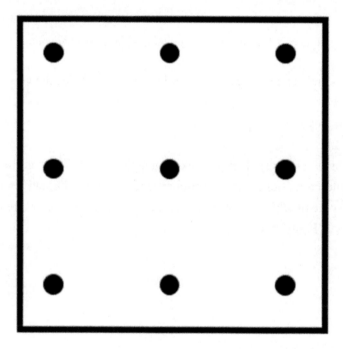

Figure 5.9. The nine-dot problem

Experiments have shown that the square box surrounding the dots is a major hindrance in finding the solution to this problem, i.e., many more people found the solution once the square was removed from the figure (Figure 5.10).

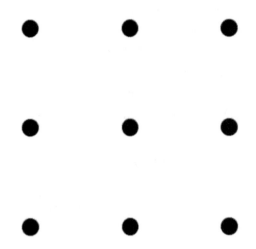

Figure 5.10. The nine-dot problem without a square box.

The reason that people find the second version easier, i.e., the version without the square box, is because the solution to this problem involves drawing lines that extend beyond the borders of this box. The solution can be found in Appendix 3.1.

This is a classical problem of thinking outside the box[126]. Over the past year, many people have looked at the problem and multiple alternatives have been proposed, some of which involved fewer than the four lines that were part of the original brief (Figure 5.11).

---

[126] Excuse me for the pun…

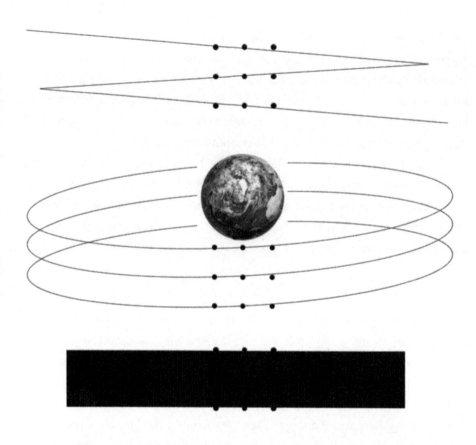

Figure 5.11. Three alternative solutions to the nine-dot problem.

Scenario planning

[Difficulty: Blue]

The objective of scenario planning is to explore the future and develop a set of innovative scenarios. The purpose of each narrative is to challenge the prevailing mindset[127]. Scenario planning involves story telling as opposed to the creation and presentation of large volumes of data. Participants are emerged in learning as the scenarios are developed. The process allows for proactive planning and helps to identify potential problems and solutions.

---

[127] Schoemaker, 1995.

Scenario planning is a creative activity, and it should be emphasised that the aim is not to predict the future[128]. The uncertainties stand next to each other as equally likely. Scenarios change several variables at the same time, without keeping others constant. It creates a narrative that are easier to grasp and use then great volumes of data. Scenario Planning protects people from overconfidence and tunnel vision in the face of uncertainty and unpredictability. The development of these scenarios requires both courage and vision.

No matter how bleak the constructed scenarios are, a set of decisions in each scenario must be internally consistent. It is almost needless to say that the tomorrow will be more uncertain and unpredictable compared to what happened today. Ultimately, it is up to you whether you are comfortable investing the time and effort in designing the processes required for Scenario Planning.

Should we think outside the box?

Iny and de Brabandere[129] argued that thinking "outside the box" is neither as desirable nor as liberating as it sounds, because the space outside the box is infinite. Faced with limitless possibilities, the human mind feels adrift and tends to fall back into the familiarity of "the box." People cannot help using mental models[130], frameworks, and theories—or, as we called them, boxes—to organize their thinking. Scenario Planning is the creation of a box, this box represents a world you have created. This world you can manipulate, mould into any shape you feel like, put away and pick it back up again free the mind to think the unthinkable.

Predicting the future of trends

The definition of the relevant time scale is of key importance. As you grow older, your value system will change. What is essential to you today might no longer be important to your future self. Change is part of life, and we tend to ignore the future rate of change. We often underestimate how much change in

---

[128] In their book *Understanding How the Future Unfolds*, Tse and Esposito (2017) explain the concept of DRIVE, which is a framework that can be applied to identify long-term trends.

[129] Iny and de Brabandere, 2010.

[130] A mental model plays a major role in cognition, reasoning and decision-making. https://en.wikipedia.org/wiki/Mental_model

our value system occurs as time elapses. The longer the period considered, the more difficult it becomes to make predictions on your future value system (see chapter *Values*).

The opposite, overpredicting, is also true. Breakthrough innovations are notoriously difficult to predict. As science progresses, most promising leads will eventually fail. Some minor progress has been made, but true breakthrough discoveries seem always just around the corner. Science is a donkey that runs forever after the carrot.

Both, the underestimation and the overprediction of trends are subject to the confirmation bias. They require a willingness to consider different scenarios to materialise.

Recognition of trends and uncertainties

Trends such as enhancing healthcare, increased incidence rates of unhealthy living, and increased awareness of the impact of unhealthy life choices can be expected to continue in the future. What is much more uncertain is the net effect of these contrary trends on the length of a human life, i.e., the future length of a healthy life is much more uncertain. In addition, the rate of medical innovation has a much higher degree of uncertainty.

Each scenario should be internally consistent in terms of fundamental trends and uncertainties.

Four conditions should be met:

Are the scenarios compelling and relevant to your situation?;
Are the scenarios internally consistent?;
Do the scenarios describe different futures rather than variations on one theme? and;
Does each scenario describe an equilibrium or a state in which the system might exist for some time?

The shrinking likelihood of a scenario

The aim of scenario planning is to create stories. In order to create believable stories, many details must be added. However, by adding more and more details, the likelihood of a given scenario to materialise becomes infinitesimal small.

171

This dynamic is elegantly illustrated by Amos Tversky's and Daniel Kahneman's Linda[131]:

Linda is 31 years old, single, outspoken, and very bright. She majored in philosophy. As a student, she was deeply concerned with issues of discrimination and social justice, and also participated in anti-nuclear demonstrations.

Which option is most likely?

Linda is a bank teller.
Linda is a bank teller and is active in the feminist movement.

Most people asked chose the second option. However, the probability of two events occurring together is always less than or equal to the probability of either one occurring itself.

Tversky and Kahneman argue that most people get this problem wrong because they rely on the representativeness heuristic. The second option seems more "representative" of Linda from the description of her, even though it is clearly mathematically less likely.

Shell and Scenario Planning

Scenario planning is the approach that Shell has used for more than half a century. In the early 1970s, scenario planning allowed Shell to prepare for an oil price shock that caused a slump in the stock market and a rise in unemployment. Due to this foresight, Shell could recover more quickly than its competitors. To this day, Shell is using scenario planning, and on the company website, one can read[132]: '[Shell] explores how the future could unfold to help people make better decisions today. By offering different possible versions of the future, our work stretches minds, confronts assumptions, and helps people think differently about the world around them. Our scenarios are not predictions about the future, do not involve a crystal ball, and are not Shell strategies. Even so, the leadership teams

---

[131] Tversky and Kahneman, 1982

[132] https://www.shell.com/energy-and-innovation/the-energy-future/scenarios/what-are-the-previous-shell-scenarios.html

at Shell have been using this work to help make decisions for more than 50 years.'

Concluding remarks: Creativity

In my view, creativity is an essential component for making high-quality decisions. Creativity is essential for imagining what could happen over the next year or during the coming decades.

The saying 'a decision can never be better than the best alternative that has been identified' is essentially a reference to creativity. Without creativity, humans simply cannot develop a set of fundamentally different and compelling alternatives. The same logic can be extended to define a comprehensive value system, a set of questions, and a series of consequences of these alternatives.

In the next chapter, we will discuss *Values*. Values define what is important to you, and values are the fundamental starting point of all decisions you will ever make.

Appendix: Solution of the nine-dot problem

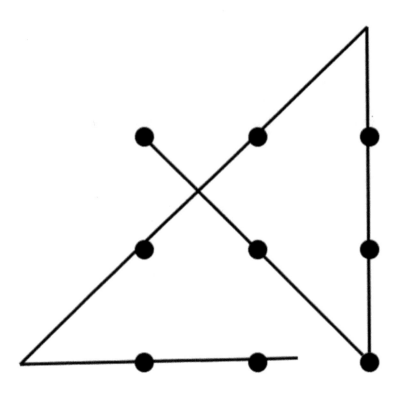

Figure 5.12. Solution to the nine-dot problem

Values

'Be brave, be curious, be determined, and overcome the odds. It can be done.'

Stephen Hawking in *Brief Answers to Big Questions*

'There are three things extremely hard: steel, a diamond, and knowing oneself.'

Benjamin Franklin

Abstract Values

Values are what we truly care about. Our decisions are the cornerstone of our existence, and our values serve as the foundation for them. Establishing one's own values requires a lot of work. The "good advice" that we receive from friends, family, co-workers, and social media affects all of us. Beware that this advice is not necessarily aligned with our personal goals. Moreover, all of us suffer from a lack of imagination.

It is difficult for us to articulate a whole set of values. Values are deeply personal and therefore very subjective. A method for defining a personal value system is the use of objective networks. Following this method, people can find a set of objectives that define the individual.

Define a personal value system

[Difficulty: Red]

Values should be the foundation of our decision-making, as values defines the meaning of life. In general, people do not spend sufficient effort finding out their personal values. If you have not defined your value system very clearly, you risk drifting between different alternatives, as the following quote from Paul Kalanithi from his book *When Breath Becomes Air* illustrates:

'The tricky part of illness is that, as you go through it, your values are constantly changing. You try to figure out what matters to you, and then you keep figuring it out. It felt like someone had taken away my credit card, and I had to learn how to budget. You may decide that you want to spend your time working as a neurosurgeon, but 2 months later, you may feel differently. Two months after that, you may want to learn to play the saxophone or devote yourself to the church.'

To me, this is a quote from a person who has not thought sufficiently about what is truly important. When reading this statement, I get a sense of a person who is drifting at sea without a North Star. The person's North Star is out of view, hiding in the mist. We all require a sense of purpose to guide us in the decisions we must make in our lives. Paul Kalanithi was intelligent enough to realise that his approach to life was not efficient, as he admits: '*You have to figure out what's most important to you.*'

Ernest Becker, in his book *The Denial of Death*, concludes: '...he has to feel and believe that what he is doing is truly heroic, timeless and supremely useful.' Becker concluded after discussing the insights of our greatest philosophers and psychologists[133] that humans want to transcend mortality by pursuing something truly meaningful, meaningful in the sense that it is fully aligned with the individual's value system.

In October 2022, my sister-in-law and I drove to the house where she grew up. Her Dad had lived in the house until he passed away the previous month. While driving, my sister-in-law made the point that life is a constant stream of choices we must make. She argued that at each decision point, there is not correct or wrong answer; the choices you make are based on your value system. Each decision involves a trade-off; you must choose between competing objectives. As long as the choice you make is aligned with your value system, it is a good choice. Life becomes very simple once you have defined your personal value system!

However, defining these personal values takes much effort. In addition to a lack of imagination (chapter *Creativity*), all of us are affected by the "good advice" offered to us by our parents, friends, social media, and colleagues. Advice on what we should aspire to can be easily obtained, but whether those views are truly consistent with what we as individuals want to achieve is a separate matter altogether. It is common for a child to choose the same profession as their parents, only to end up deeply frustrated later in life. People are influenced by Instagram©, TikTok© and LinkedIn©. Not realising that the views

---

[133] E.g., Freud, Jung, Kierkegaard, Rank, Nietzsche

in many posts are not reality – each of us is wearing a mask that hides our true personality.

It requires commitment to expose the personal values that defines you as a person. It takes effort to clear the mist. Finding direction in your life – defining the aims of your life, how to define your calling, and fine-tuning your internal guidance system – requires continuous learning and reassessment, and you will find many obstacles along the way. You will be faced with doubt and distraction. You will feel insecure, stressed, bored, and might even be exposed to depression (e.g., midlife life crises). Regardless of how difficult it is, it is worth the effort because if you have not defined what is truly important to you, you will likely make the wrong choices in life.

The four questions to ask yourself

Atul Gawande in his book *Being Mortal*, states: '[The patient] had, I estimated for her, a 75 % chance I'd make her future better, at least for a little while, and a 25 % chance I'd make it worse. So, what then was the right thing for her to do? Why was the choice so agonising? The choice, I realised, was far more complicated than the risk calculation. For how you weigh relief from nausea, and the chances of being able to eat again, against the possibilities of pain, of infections, of having to live with stooling into a bag.'

Atul continues: '[Doctors have] been wrong about what our job is in medicine. We think our job is to ensure health and survival. But really, it is larger than that. It enables well-being. Well-being is about the reasons one wishes to be alive. Those reasons matter not just at the end of life, or when debility comes, but all along the way.'

Atul subsequently defined four key questions:

What is your understanding of your situation and its potential outcomes?;
What are your fears and what are your hopes?;
What are the trade-offs you are willing to make and not willing to make?;
What is the course of action that best serves this understanding?

Subjectivity of values

[Difficulty: Blue]

Just imagine that tomorrow morning you find out that you have an additional 4 months to live. How would you spend that time? Would you watch television, climb Mount Everest, or spend these final months with your family? Clearly, all these options have a different personal appeal to the individual. Is climbing Mt Everest more or less important to you than spending more time with your family?

In July 2022, I lost most of my hair. The fact that I was almost completely bald was irrelevant to me. In contrast, a family member who has been diagnosed with pancreatic cancer told me that the only thing she could remember from the conversation with her doctor was that she would lose her hair. Clearly, the impact of losing her hair is much larger to her than it is for me.

The subjective nature of personal benefits, on how to spend the final months of your life, and the importance of hair loss have a pronounced implication on decision making. These differences in personal benefits are rooted in your personal value system.

The benefit is referred to as a utility. Utility is intimately connected to your value system. The higher the utility of a given choice, the more it contributes to the achievement of your fundamental objective. Your choice will have a massive impact on your realised Quality of Life.

Personal values are deeply personal. Therefore, a "bad choice" might simply reflect a different value system. This decision might be completely consistent with someone else's values, even though we might not agree with it. It is a common error to impose our value system on someone else. Hence, we cannot understand why they make a different choice when presented with the same facts.

A Clash of Value Systems

In early March 2023, I travelled to Berlin to meet a friend. This friend happened to be the best man at our wedding. After a couple of years in Copenhagen, we separated, and he has been living in Germany for more than twenty years before we rekindled our friendship.

We were sitting in a bar when I pointed out a small Vietnamese restaurant just across the street and suggested we have dinner there. My friend looked at me in shock – how could I suggest where to eat without having conducted some prior research? He got out his phone and searched restaurants in the part of Berlin where we were and started looking at people's reviews of various alternative places to have a bite to eat. I realised that this was a clash of personal value systems! For my friend, it is really important that the food he eats is as good as it possibly can be. For me, on the other hand, it is much more important to have easy choices – the Vietnamese restaurant was located about ten metres from the spot where we are having our beers. However, I do have another core value; I want to please my friends, and that is why I did not mind walking for twenty-five minutes in the cold Berlin winter weather to reach a restaurant he approved upon. There is an additional reason why I believe that the probability is low that the restaurant would serve low-quality food. I believe that the market for restaurants is highly efficient. Many restaurants go bankrupt in the first couple of years after opening. Apparently, 65% of restaurants had to close their doors in the UK over the past 12 months[134].

Exploring different value systems

I conducted a series of interviews in which I asked participants to place in order a set of cards with various statements that were related to their value system (Table 2.1). The order of these statements provides insight into what matters most and what statement is completely irrelevant to the participants.

The statements in Table 2.1 are ordered by decreasing average values. *Family* is judged to be the most important value by all subjects, except Subject F, who scores *Health* as the most important. I find it very interesting to see that Subjects A and B, who both have terminal cancer, scored Health below or *on par* with 7 (Subject A) and 10 (Subject B) different personal values.

Another intriguing finding is that, in addition to *Family, Independence, Freedom of choice, Honesty, and Reliability* received higher average scores than *Health*[135].

Personally, I am of the opinion that *Acquiring knowledge* is crucial to me. I am surprising that this value is not valued as much by my fellow subjects. Only Subject C shared this value with me, and the others ranked this value at the bottom of their list.

These statements can be interpreted in many ways. For example, the word *Nature* is interpreted by some people as a beautiful landscape, or it can represent an ecosystem on which humans rely for their survival, or it can even mean God. For some people, there are multiple terms that they perceive to be synonyms. For

---

[134]https://www.bighospitality.co.uk/Article/2023/01/31/The-number-of-restaurant-businesses-going-bust-has-leapt-65-to-the-highest-level-in-more-than-a-decade
[135] I do realise that I only obtained data on eight subjects – no I am not making a statistical claim here.

example, *Honesty, Reliability* and *Respect,* could be interpreted as meaning the same thing.

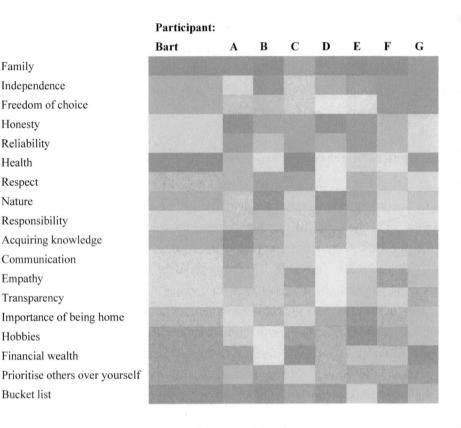

| | Participant: | | | | | | |
	Bart	**A**	**B**	**C**	**D**	**E**	**F**	**G**
Family								
Independence								
Freedom of choice								
Honesty								
Reliability								
Health								
Respect								
Nature								
Responsibility								
Acquiring knowledge								
Communication								
Empathy								
Transparency								
Importance of being home								
Hobbies								
Financial wealth								
Prioritise others over yourself								
Bucket list								

Table 2.1. A group of people with value systems.

As we grow up and get older, our value system changes. I made an assessment of how my personal value changed over the years (Table 2.2). As you can see *Family* was not always in the top spot. When I was in my twenties and forties, *Independence* and *Freedom of choice* were more important to me. Also note that when I was in my forties, I had a young family, and I was working very hard on my career. *Financial wealth* was much more important to me at that stage in my life. Although Bucket list not very important to me at present, it was much more important when I was in my tens and twenties[136].

---

[136] Tintin was one of my childhood heroes!

	Participant:			
	Bart at 10	**Bart at 20**	**Bart at 40**	**Bart at 53**
Independence				
Freedom of choice				
Family				
Nature				
Acquiring knowledge				
Health				
Responsibility				
Respect				
Honesty				
Reliability				
Communication				
Bucket list				
Transparency				
Empathy				
Financial wealth				
Importance of being home				
Hobbies				
Prioritise others over yourself				

Table 2.2 Changing values throughout my life.

Now that we have established that our value system is changing during our life, we face an immediate dilemma; the choices you make in the next stage of your life will those choices be aligned with your future value system. For example, consider retirement choices. You have a busy career, and at some stage you will stop working, and you will have loads of spare time. This is the time to pursue hobbies for which you never had time for, because before you were pursuing your career. However, these hobbies might not live up to your expectation – these hobbies might disappoint. They might simply not be as much fun as you currently believe they would be, and your value system might have changed[137].

After my first operation I decided that I would not have a second operation. I was convinced that I would not have a second brain operation, but when the

---

[137] I used AI to complete my writing. See 'Appendix: AI and writing' for details.

moment was there, I changed my mind. I decided to go ahead with the operation anyway…

Reverting to happiness baseline

How would you feel if I told you that you just had won the lottery? Or you found out that instead of having a couple more months to live, you learned that you were cancer free? Or something else happened that makes you feel ecstatic? In those cases, would it be possible to be happier than your normal degree of happiness? How long would it take to revert to your happiness baseline? What if a second event occurred, e.g., a second case of a terminal illness? Do we all have the same happiness baseline or is there a range of happiness baseline levels?

After I learned that I had a Glioblastoma it took me 8 months to get back to my former self. Eight months, from the 26th of April 2022 to the 17th of January 2023, were needed before I was able to cope with the knowledge that I had a brain tumour. I had spent eight months drowned in noise, it took eight months before the horrible, horrendous, noises were gone. I don't know whether these eight months are generally applicable, but what I do know is that this experience left me with some very deep, painful, scars.

I know that this experience is the most traumatic event I have ever lived through. Hence, all other events – positive or negative – should have a shorter impact duration. For example, when I was awarded my bonus in February 2023, it hardly affected my happiness. Although the bonus was a substantial amount of money it did not increase my happiness much. In the end that money was used to pay for a safari in Tanzania, but even that experience increased my happiness for only a short while. In terms of happiness, the impact of that holiday paled in comparison to the diagnoses of my illness.

I belief that even if one of my children, my wife or me would be affected by another terminal illness, it would be easier to cope with. It remains to be seen how much easier such experience would be. But I do realise if such event were to occur that the fact that I had to live through these eight months will help to get to grips with such future event.

Objective network

[Difficulty: Red]

Value-focused thinking differs from other decision-making approaches in that it emphasizes the importance of identifying and articulating fundamental values before focusing on identifying alternatives. People tend to focus first on identifying alternatives rather than on articulating values. Keeney recognises that decision makers are typically faced with incomplete information and these decision makers cannot evaluate all alternatives. Value-focused thinking recognizes these limitations and provides a framework for decision-making that is more flexible and adaptable to real-world situations. The general methodology developed by Ralph Keeney[138] creates a structure for these objectives, known as an *objective network*. The purpose of an objective network is to clearly articulate a hierarchy of objectives that allows decision makers to identify value trade-offs[139].

Core benefits of objective networks:

Create insight by structuring a value framework;
Recognise objectives either as *means-to-an-end* or *strategic*;
Define measurable attributes for means-to-end objectives.

Detailed functioning of an objective network

When thinking about objectives, one can recognise a hierarchy of objectives; not all objectives are of equal importance. The process of recognising a hierarchical structure amongst the objectives provides clarity, deepens your insight into the decision problem, and clarifies the distinction between strategic objectives and means-to-end based objectives.

Value-focussed thinking forces participants to prioritise values, which are the principles used in an evaluation. The values, or objectives, labelled "strategic" have an intrinsic value because these are the objectives we truly care about. These objectives can include ethical principles. I have identified *maximise happiness* as my personal *strategic objective*. Many organisations have developed sets of core values that provide a set of guiding principles to all their

---

[138] Keeney, 1992.

[139] Keeney distinguishes between strategic and fundamental objectives. Fundamental objectives are a subset of strategic objectives and are selected because they are relevant for a given decision. For example, imagine a situation where you have an accident and need to go to the hospital as quickly as possible. The sole relevant objective in this situation is to get medical attention as quickly as possible; none of the other fundamental objectives will feature in your decision. In this situation, you do not really care about maximising "freedom of choice" or "worthwhile activities".

employees. Many pharmaceutical companies have adopted the core objective that we should look after our patients. *Means-to-end objectives* have no intrinsic values. The purpose of means-to-an-end objectives is to link strategic objectives to attributes that can be measured.

Once the means-to-an-end objectives have been recognised, it is feasible to develop an attribute or several attributes that quantifies the means-to-an-end objective, i.e., attributes make a means-to-an-end objectives countable. These attributes allow a decision maker to assess the value of a decision. A comparison of the values of different choices enables the decision maker to create a rich set of insights into a complex situation in a way that complements intuitive thinking.

Keeney's personal strategic objective network

Ralph L. Keeney's personal strategic objective network is shown in Figure 6.1. Keeney's strategic objective *Maximise Happiness,* shown in the right-most box, represents the most fundamental strategic objective. The choices and actions made ultimately impact *Happiness.* Keeney wrote, 'I believe society should provide opportunities for individuals to have a good quality of life and I would like to contribute to society to maintain and improve its opportunities.'

Apart from Maximise Happiness, all other boxes are examples of means-to-end objectives. The term "worthwhile" is used to indicate how well the activities and relationships facilitate usefulness in achieving strategic objectives. To pursue anything, one needs the opportunity and freedom to pursue it. Keeney introduced, on the left side of the diagram, the boxes *To minimise constraints on freedom of choice* and *To minimise constraints on opportunities for choice.* In his book, Keeney provides several examples of how the insights obtained through this model have guided him in his decision-making, including his experiences while writing his book *Value Focussed Thinking.*

On the upper left of the diagram, there is a box labelled *To minimise constraints on freedom of choice.* Inside this box, you will find the following: Maximise health, Maximise financial wellbeing and Maximise available time. We can measure all three objectives. One could measure someone's health by employing a large range of biomarkers, such as cholesterol levels for cardio fitness, changes in PSA values for one's risk of prostate cancer, and an examination of the blood vessels to assess the likelihood of developing diabetes. Likewise, an assessment can be made to test your financial wellbeing by looking at your pension savings and by tracking the number of meetings you have in your diary. Finally, an assessment can be made on how busy your schedule is; ask yourself would I have the bandwidth to take on such-and-such task?

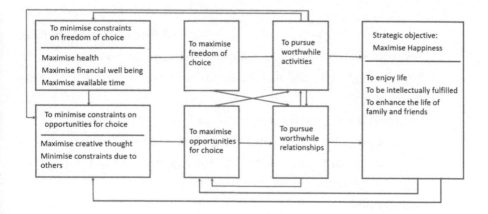

Figure 6.1. Ralph Keeney's personal objective network.

The two arrows at the bottom of the figure (those that originate from the strategic objective) represent a feedback loop, i.e., they have an impact on the next decision that is assessed in this framework.

I have adapted this diagram to my personal needs in the chapter *Surviving*.

Concluding remarks: Values

All choices are good if they are consistent with the decision maker's value system. Value systems are very personal. Individuals have unique value systems – all of which have a different set of values.

No value system is defined by a single factor; instead, there are many aspects that determine your set of values. Defining a value system is not easy. Much effort is required to define a personal value system.

The methods that can be used to assess a value system are discussed in the next section – Decision analysis.

Appendix: AI and writing

During the time I have written my book, AI has revolutionised writing. By the time I had completed the fourth draft of my manuscript in November 2023, there were already many options available to me. I submitted the entire book to

Trinka[140]. I used an AI to ensure that there were no spelling or grammar errors in the text I had written.

A couple of days later, I fed ChatGPT the bullets as shown below:

In the early 1990s, I was conducting geological fieldwork in Marble Bar;
I investigated the fossilised remains of Archaean stromatolites;
Once the fieldwork was finished we visited Shark Bay to look at living stromatolites;
Darwinian life was established as far back as 4 billion years ago;
Charles Lyell's famous maxim, 'the present is the key to the past';
Max Tegmark in Life 3.0 states that the objective of life is defined by the laws of physics;
Goal oriented;
Reflections on my personal value system;
In 2023 I have a very different value system.

After feeding the AI this information, I received a coherent story featuring all information I mentioned in these bullets.

'Marble Bar, located in Western Australia's Pilbara region, is indeed a geological treasure trove. Scientists have been delving into its ancient granite rocks to unravel the mysteries of Earth's origins. These rocks near Marble Bar provide insights into how water entered Earth's deepest crust from the mantle below, shaping the continents nearly four billion years ago. The unique geological patterns in the Pilbara region hint at something fundamentally different that occurred early in our planet's history.

But that's not all! The Pilbara rocks also harbor records of our planet's first lifeforms. The stromatolite rock formations found across the Pilbara, including those in Shark Bay, house both living and fossilized microbialites. These tiny microbes offer glimpses into the earliest microscopic signs of life on Earth, spanning an impressive 3.5 billion years of antiquity. Imagine the scale of existence they represent in the context of life as we understand it today.

Speaking of Shark Bay, it's one of only two places globally where living marine stromatolites exist. These ancient structures provide a window into what life on Earth was like 3.5 billion years ago. Consider them living fossils—the

---

[140] www.cloud.trinka.ai

earliest record of life on our planet. These stromatolites thrive in Hamelin Pool, where the extreme salinity and unique underwater landscape create an environment that echoes our distant past.

So, from the ancient granite rocks of Marble Bar to the living stromatolites of Shark Bay, these geological wonders remind us that the present truly holds the key to understanding our planet's past. And as for value systems, well, they can evolve just like our understanding of Earth's history!'

Underneath the text I found three questions and once I clicked on the question: 'How does AI relate to life's objective?' The following text appeared:

'Artificial Intelligence (AI), like life itself, is intricately woven into the fabric of the universe. Let's explore this connection:

1. *The Cosmic Algorithm:*
   Physicists have discovered that all laws of classical physics can be mathematically reformulated in an analogous way: out of all ways that nature could choose to do something, it offers the optimal way, which typically boils down to minimizing or maximizing some quantity. If a person is trying to optimize something (for example, their score, wealth, or happiness), we naturally describe their pursuit of it as goal-oriented. So if nature itself is trying to optimize something, then no wonder that goal-oriented behavior can emerge: it was hardwired in from the start, in the very laws of physics.
   Max Tegmark, in his book "Life 3.0", argues that the objective of life is defined by the laws of physics. The goal of life, according to Tegmark, is to extract as much energy as possible from its environment. A great way to achieve this goal is to make copies of itself—hence the emergence of Darwinian life as far back as 4 billion years ago.
2. *Optimization and Emergence:*
   Optimization is a fundamental property of life. From the smallest cells to complex organisms, life seeks efficiency, adaptation, and survival. Whether it's a plant turning toward sunlight or a predator tracking its prey, optimization is the silent conductor of life's symphony.
   AI, too, mirrors this optimization. Machine learning algorithms optimize parameters to minimize error or maximize accuracy. Neural networks

evolve through training, adapting to patterns in data. The emergence of intelligence from these algorithms echoes life's quest for efficiency.

3. *The Campfire of Consciousness:*

   Imagine a campfire—a gathering of minds sharing stories, warmth, and dreams. Our consciousness, too, emerges from the cosmic fire. We optimize our experiences, seeking joy, connection, and purpose.

   AI, in its nascent form, mimics this campfire. It learns, adapts, and optimizes. Its objective? To solve problems, assist us, and perhaps—like the stromatolites of old—shape the future.

4. *Reflections on Values:*

   As for personal value systems, they evolve. In 2023, my values may differ significantly from earlier years. Adventure, collaboration, creativity— they shape our decisions. But perhaps the most profound value is family—the bonds that transcend time and algorithms.

   Independence, too, holds sway. The desire to explore, question, and forge our own path—whether as humans or AI.

   In this dance of optimization, let us celebrate both the ancient stromatolites and the neural networks. For life, in all its forms, seeks meaning, connection, and the warmth of shared existence.'

…woah…that is frightening and impressive at the same time…

AI is revolutionising writing. I struggle to see where this development is taking mankind. It is simply too easy to write a couple of bullets and let AI do the hard work of writing a story.

Decision Analysis

'I listened in quiet awe as a paediatric neurosurgeon…delivered the clinical facts as well, acknowledging the tragedy of the situation…[the surgeon described] the planned operation, the likely outcomes and possibilities, what decisions needed to be made now, what decisions they started thinking about but did need to decide on immediately and sorts of decisions they shouldn't worry about all yet…I feared I was losing sight of the singular importance of human relationships, not between patients and their families but between doctor and patient….my highest ideal was not saving lives – everyone dies eventually – but guiding a patient or family to an understanding of death or illness.'

Paul Kalanithi in *When Breath Becomes Air*

'I found it rather difficult to follow the complex plot [of Godzilla]. All my pieces of skull were loose and being rattled around by the surround sound.'

Adam Blain in *Pear Shaped*

'The choices don't stop, however. Life is a choice, and they are relentless. No sooner have made one choice than another is upon you.'

Atul Gawande in *Being Mortal*

Abstract Decision Analysis

Decision analysis is a communication toolkit. Each tool serves a different purpose. The old saying "the perfect hammer makes a poor saw" very much applies. Of particular importance are: 1) assessing the quality of a decision, 2) making difficult trade-offs, and 3) ensuring that our analysis addresses the right problem.

Decision Quality is a checklist consisting of six dimensions. Before committing to any decision, the decision-maker should make a conscious

189

evaluation of all dimensions. Decision Quality is the only chance you have as a decision maker to improve the probability of ultimately ending up in a desirable situation.

A common decision challenge for people is selecting their preference from a set of alternatives. Humans typically do not have the discipline to handle multiple criteria consistently and are prone to "decision fatigue". When a decision maker is faced with many alternatives and conflicting criteria, *Multi-Criteria Decision Analysis* provides structure and process.

Decision analysis starts by identifying the problem that needs to be solved. A well-developed definition of what is in scope and what is outside the scope of decision is the most important and hardest aspect of decision analysis to get right. The definition of the decision problem is referred to as the *Frame*. Remember that once a decision is made, the effort you invested in making the analysis is irretrievably lost. Therefore, we better ensure that the frame is appropriate.

Other techniques that are discussed are: *Influence diagrams, Decision trees,* and *Strategy tables*. In the concluding section of this chapter, it will be illustrated how a wholistic framework can be developed based on these six methodologies.

Frame

[Difficulty: Blue]

The first step in decision analysis is to define the overall problem to be solved. What is in the scope and what is out of the scope of the decision to be made? This step is referred to as the development of a *frame*. In my professional experience, a well-developed frame is the most important and hardest aspect of decision analysis to achieve. Developing an appropriate frame is all about patience – people tend to be so eager to act that they simply forget to pause and think. A perfect model is useless if it addresses the wrong question. Remember that once a decision is made, the effort you invested in making the analysis is irretrievably lost. Therefore, we better ensure that the frame is appropriate.

To develop a frame, a clear problem statement is needed. What is the problem to be solved? What are the decision criteria, i.e., what conditions must be satisfied for the decision to be optimal? Is the decision hierarchy clear, i.e., do all stakeholders agree on 1) what decisions have been made, 2) what decision has the current focus, and 3) what decisions can be made later?

Core benefits of a well-developed frame:

Pool the knowledge of key stakeholders and experts;
Generate a common understanding of the decision situation (including timelines, i.e., how far into the future should the frame extend).

The art of framing

A frame that is too broad risks involving too much detail, can be overwhelming, and can lead to paralysis by analysis. A frame that is too narrow risks failing to identify all relevant uncertainties and decisions. Therefore, a narrow frame risk missing opportunities to mitigate negative consequences. People tend to create frames that are too narrow.

The cartoon below illustrates the need for an appropriate frame (Figure 7.1). The overall problem is to assess the safety of the boat. The panel on the left depicts a frame that is too broad. Its landscape depicts a mountain range, a river, and a forest, but there is no sign of a boat. The panel on the right depicts a frame that is too narrow. It shows an occupied boat that is drifting down the river, but it fails to show the portion of the river that the boat will shortly enter. The panel in the centre illustrates the correct frame, as it depicts the waterfall and rocks that the boat is approaching.

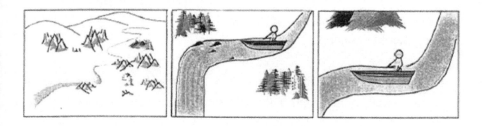

Figure 7.1. Development of an appropriate frame. The waterfall and rocks are the key issues that the analysis should capture and are visible only in the centre panel.

To be effective, the frame must focus on establishing the scope of the problem. Therefore, the frame should not attempt to address ambitious goals, such as the following:

- Create a detailed plan of all planned activities;
- Identify an extensive list of all uncertainties;
- Answer all the questions and issues raised.

Detailed workings of an opportunity statement

How do you write an opportunity statement[141]? When do you write it and when should you update the opportunity statement?

An opportunity statement should be revised once the existing opportunity statement has lost its relevance. New information has arisen, uncertainties have been resolved, or decisions have been made, making the existing opportunity statement obsolete. An existing opportunity statement needs to be revised once it has lost some, or all its, value.

An opportunity statement should be concise and clear. I have spent much of my career rewriting draft opportunity statements. Many people struggle with clearly expressing themselves and often use woolly grammar and their sentences lack a clear focus. Take a look at the following opportunity statement:

'I have a strong desire to remain fit and keep up with my daily activities for as long as possible. Although at present it is unknown what the future holds, I hope to achieve this by doing lots of exercise and having a long sleep each night. I might have to adapt my lifestyle if I become too fatigued to maintain my current level of performance. In this scenario, I will have to resort to an early afternoon sleep.'

First, this opportunity statement is way too long. It is possible to greatly reduce the length of the text. The opportunity statement starts with a value statement: 'I have a strong desire to remain fit' I would recommend making this statement a bit more general and stating something like 'Quality of Life is important to me.' I would also recommend deleting the subordinate clause: 'and keep up with my daily activities for as long as possible.' The start of the next sentence: 'Although at present it is unknown what the future holds' does not convey any relevant information; therefore, this sentence can also be deleted. The remainder of the sentence: 'I hope to achieve this by doing lots of exercise

---

[141] An "opportunity statement" should not be confused with a "fundamental objective". The concepts of fundamental objectives are described in the chapter *Values*.

and having long sleep each night' talks about a planned activity. The planned activities should not be included in an opportunity statement. Therefore, this can be deleted too. The following two sentences: 'I might have to adapt my lifestyle if I get too fatigued to maintain my current level of performance. In this scenario, I will have to resort to an early afternoon sleep.' It also lists a possible outcome and a mechanism to deal with it. I would recommend using the following opportunity statement:

'I want to explore activities that result in a high Quality of Life.'

Influence Diagram

[Difficulty: Green]

'I have so much to do! And there's so little time!'

John Gunther, Jr. in *Death be not Proud.*

In an *influence diagram*, we capture issues and categorise them as one of the following:

- Givens;
- Uncertainties;
- Decisions.

An influence diagram is my personal default choice for starting an analysis. An influence diagram allows people to create a structure around a decision. Decisions come in an infinite number of different shapes and forms. In many cases, the decision is not well defined and typically requires some boundaries and structure.

An influence diagram is a perfect tool for brainstorming sessions. Participants can simply call out *issues*. Calling out these issues is a useful exercise as participants are forced to express each issue using succinct and comprehensible language. In my professional experience, the process of building an influence diagram is an effective way to detect double entries of issues. It is common for people to use different formulations for the same issue. Each of these issues can be categorised as an *uncertainty*, a *decision*, or a *given*. *Givens* are facts that must be considered. Often the givens are resolved uncertainties or decisions already taken. The point in calling them out explicitly is that it removes

193

any ambiguity about the current status of the uncertainties and decisions, i.e., are they a given or still uncertain or to be decided?

Uncertainties and decisions come in two types: those that are "relevant for now" and those that are "relevant for later"[142]. Only those that are labelled "relevant for now" will be taken forward in the next step of the analysis.

Core benefits of influence diagrams:

Gather all issues[143] relevant to the analysis;

Create a list of key decisions;

Alignment of facts, uncertainties, and decisions;

A visual method to develop a one-page model.

It is important to note that the influence diagrams described above are not used to develop a Bayesian Network. The theory of Bayesian Networks goes beyond the scope of this book. Readers interested in Bayesian Networks are referred to Owens et al. (1997).

Detailed workings of the influence diagram

One important aspect to note is that a decision situation continuously evolves over time. As more information is gathered some uncertainties get resolved. Decisions are taken and their associated choices disappear.

I have found the influence diagram to be ideal for starting an analysis because it facilitates brainstorming. A participant can simply call out a potential *issue*, which the team would then categorise as – an uncertainty, a decision, or a given. It is common that some discussion is needed to identify the correct category of an issue. For example, there might be some confusion amongst team members about whether an uncertainty has been resolved and therefore should be categorised as a *given*. One of the virtues of an influence diagram is that the mere act of constructing it will aid the experts in their understanding of the decision.

---

[142] This two-fold distinction between "relevant for now" and "relevant for later" is shared with the decision hierarchy method (see Communication chapter).

[143] Issues are considerations or factors in the context of the decision.

An influence diagram[144] uses arrows to depict the dependencies among the givens (i.e., facts, solid assumptions). Many of the givens are uncertainties that have been resolved or decisions that have been made. The optimal choice might be dependent on the outcome of an uncertainty.

Below is an example of an influence diagram. The three types of issue are depicted as follows: givens are represented by diamonds; uncertainties are shown as rectangles with rounded corners and decisions appear as rectangles with square corners[145]. The diagram shows four *givens*: "Tumour will be removed", "Presence of brain tumour", "Large uncertainty will persist" and "Hospital is world class". There are six uncertainties shown "for now" as ovals: "What are our decisions", "Outcome biopsy", "Long term prognosis", "Quality of Life during treatment", "Long term prognosis" and "Happiness". Two uncertainties "for later": "Other available treatments" and "Outcome second brain operation". Three decisions "for now": "Clinical studies", "Treatment post operation", "Prioritisation of tasks" and a single decision "for later": "Retrieving driving license".

Arrows indicate relationships in the diagram. One can identify the logical sequences of nodes. For example, from the given "Tumour will be removed", via the uncertainties: "Outcome biopsy", "Long term prognosis" to finally a decision on the "Prioritisation of tasks". During the operation, a biopsy will be taken that provides information on the long-term prognosis that is informative on the Quality of Life. Once uncertainty around the Quality of Life is resolved, a decision can be made on how the tasks can be prioritised (see decision tree for Tasks; Figure 7.2)

---

[144] For additional information on influence diagrams, the reader can refer to Howard (1989, 1990).

[145] I used the basic functionality of PowerPoint to draw this influence diagram but drawing them manually would often suffice.

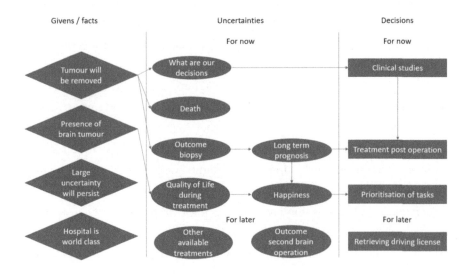

| Givens / facts | Uncertainties | Decisions |

Figure 7.2. Influence diagram listing givens, uncertainties and decisions.

Ever since I was diagnosed with brain cancer, I have been periodically updating my influence diagram. The version shown in Figure 7.2 was up to date before my operation on May 30, 2022. At the time, the biopsy result was uncertain. In the next version of the influence diagram, the uncertainty around the biopsy result was resolved and a long-term prognosis was made. The uncertainty around the long-term prognosis was identified as a *given*. The influence diagram requires updating each time additional, reliable information becomes available.

Decision Tree

[Difficulty: Red]

Decision trees are diagrams that provide structure to a decision problem. A decision tree is an excellent tool for communicating the rationale motivating a decision. A well-drawn decision tree can convey a convincing message on the impact of uncertainties and trade-offs occurring at some point in the future as well as explore options around medical treatment. A decision tree can be used to determine an expected value, i.e., the "average"[146] benefit that you can expect to obtain.

Core benefits of Decision Trees:

A fast method to create deep insight;

Definition of scenarios following the resolution of uncertainties and choices of decisions;

Time sequence of uncertainties and decisions;

A visual method to develop a one-page model.

Detailed workings of the decision tree

Decision trees[147] visualise four elements: uncertainty-nodes, decisions-nodes, end-nodes and time. Time is generally encoded from left to right, and the sequence of uncertainty-nodes and decision-nodes reflect the relative timing of events. Each of the end-nodes represents a single scenario. A scenario is a unique combination of decisions made and a set of outcomes of all uncertainties that lead to a specific end-node.

A decision-node represents a set of choices available to a decision maker at a given point in time. The logic for a decision tree is very simple; select the option that is best aligned with your objective. Future decision points are typically preceded by an uncertainty-node.

Uncertainty-nodes consist of a discrete set of outcomes, typically four or fewer, that are probability-weighted (i.e., a probability has been assigned to each of the scenarios and the sum of the probabilities should add up to 100%). The outcomes should be mutually exclusive (i.e., no overlap between the scenarios is allowed).

The workings of a decision tree are illustrated by the example shown in Figure 7.3. The first node in the tree is an uncertainty node. There are two

---

[146] The expected number when rolling a die is 3.5. This value is not feasible. A similar scenario holds for the expected value obtained by solving a decision tree. There may not be a scenario that has a corresponding value to the expected value.

[147] Many good books have been written about decision trees, such as Hammond, Keeney and Raiffa (1999), Clemen and Reilly (2001), Goodwin and Wright (2004), McNamee and Celona (2005) and Bratvold and Begg (2010). This literature provides additional insight into the consequences and trade-offs between multiple measures, the value of flexibility, and risk attitudes.

possible outcomes for the "Remaining time Quality of Life is 100%", "More than a month" and "Less than a month". The first alternative has a probability of 75% and the second alternative has a probability of 25%. The total must be added to 100%. The second node is an example of the decision node called "Task". There are three alternatives to choose from: "Family, writing, work, walking, cycling", "Family, writing, walking" and "Family". The choice made at a decision node is conditional on the uncertainties resolved and decisions made. In the scenario where there is "more than a month of 100% Quality of Life remaining", the optimal choice is "Family, writing, work, walking, cycling". In the alternative scenario, "Less than a month", the preference switches to "Family". Preferences are indicated by a bold arrow. In this decision tree, a total of six unique outcomes are possible.

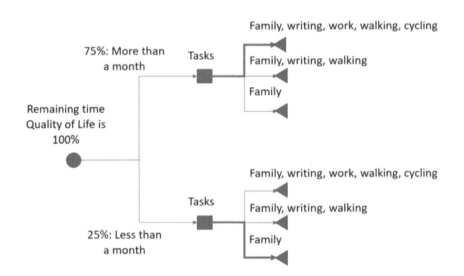

Figure 7.3. An example of a decision tree.

One must be careful to ensure that the decision trees do not grow too big. An unwieldy decision tree is not useful because cluttering will prevent clear communication. A technique that can be used to summarise a decision tree is to simply list all uncertainties and decisions, with all their outcomes in the order of occurrence, as shown in Figure 7.4. The decision tree shown in Figure 7.4 has 4*4*4 = 64 outcomes.

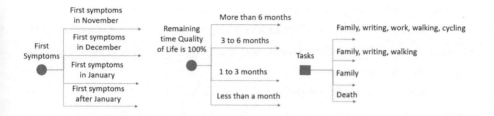

Figure 7.4. Shorthand notation of a decision tree.

The expected value is not a sensible metric to calculate in the decision trees in Figure 7.3 and Figure 7.4. Although one could develop a utility metric that is reflective of the perceived benefit of a given outcome, I am not convinced that this would add any insight to this analysis. In the section *Surviving,* a decision tree is developed that investigates the overall survival time. In this situation, it makes sense to determine the duration of overall survival.

The worth of a decision tree is quantified by its expected value. The expected is normally expressed as a monetary value, i.e., millions of pounds. But this is not necessarily true, in this situation it is more appropriate to express the value of the tree as "months to live." The expected value is determined using a rollback procedure. The logic of this procedure is that one starts at the far right of the decision tree. For decision nodes, one simply takes the branch with the highest utility score and disregards all other branches. For uncertainty nodes, we calculate the probability-weighted average by taking the total of products. In other words, we calculate the summed product of the probabilities and the utility of all scenarios.

Influence diagrams can be redrawn as decision trees. Both influence diagrams and decision trees contain uncertainties and decisions nodes. Drawing a decision tree is much harder than drawing an influence diagram because decision trees require a definition of the possible outcomes for each uncertainty and the choices for each decision.

Strategy tables

[Difficulty: Red]

Good decision making implies a choice between a set of alternatives, not a binary choice between the acceptance or rejection of a proposal. It is worth the time and effort to create a rich set of distinct, compelling, alternatives. A decision cannot be better than the best alternative that has been identified.

The process of working through a *strategy table* facilitates collaboration between the patient and their family and medical staff to reflect on the problem in a structured manner.

Strategy tables enable experts to break down a decision into its parts. The process of dividing, splitting the problem into smaller, more understandable parts is helpful as it enables all stakeholders to contribute to the bigger picture.

A strategy table is a graphical tool that matches strategies to a set of choices for a series of decisions. The process to follow is selecting a certain strategy and asking yourself which of the listed options would best support the realisation of that strategy.

The result of the exercise is a one-page summary of the different strategies and choices available. This process allows the patient to evaluate whether the proposed alternatives are fundamentally different as each alternative should have a unique set of choices.

Core benefits of strategy tables:

Facilitates the development of truly distinct options;
Allows us to think about strategies and decisions separately;
Allows us to think about choices for each decision separately.

Detailed workings of the strategy table

In the first column of the strategy table, different alternatives are listed. Alternatives are referred to as *strategies* in the context of a strategy table. One must be mindful that these alternatives should be do-able, compelling, and truly distinct. The development of a good set of alternatives requires commitment from all stakeholders.

The remaining columns are used for decisions and choices. Decisions can be added to the top column of the table. The possible choices are listed below the question. Finally, we can complete the strategy table. For each strategy, we select the optimal set of choices for each question listed. In case one ends up with two identical set of choices one should wonder whether you have not pursued a single objective through two different routes. Ask yourself are these two strategies truly distinct? How can I make these two strategies different? Figure 7.5 shows a strategy table that analyses three strategies: *Maximise Quality of Life, Balancing Quality of Life and length of life*, and *Maximise length of life*.

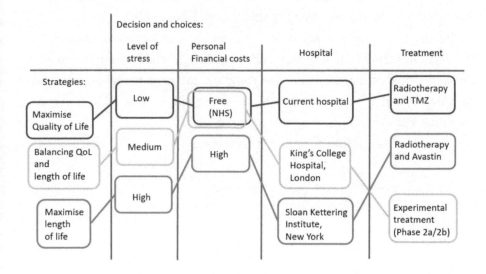

Figure 7.5. An example of a strategy table focussing on three strategies and four decisions.

Over years, I have noticed that many people struggle with the creation of meaningful labels, i.e., short descriptions that are clear and non-confusing. I can advise you to simply use numbers in the strategy table and add a longer description of the alternative underneath the table.

Multi-Criteria Decision Analysis

[Difficulty: Red]

'There is no moment for which we cannot be grateful because in every moment, even difficult ones, we have the opportunity to something.'

Brother David Steindl-Rast, TED

A common decision challenge for people is selecting their preference from a set of alternatives. *Multi-Criteria Decision Analysis* (MCDA) is a powerful approach for identifying your preferred choice by clearly articulating the trade-offs that exist for multiple criteria. Human decision makers typically do not have the discipline to handle multiple criteria in a consistent way and are prone to *decision fatigue*. MCDA provides structure and process when a decision maker

201

is faced with many alternatives and conflicting criteria. MCDA facilitates a rigorous quantification of preferences for a single criterion and across different criteria. MCDA helps the decision maker to establish decision criteria, prioritise those decision criteria, and rank the alternatives accordingly.

Below is an illustration of how to select your preferred clinical trial; however, this approach is completely generic and can be applied to many decision problems. For example, one could use the same model to gain insight on which treatment to take or how to select the activity you want to pursue in your final years.

Core benefits of Multi-Criteria Decision Analysis:

Internal consistency and logical soundness;
Transparency and ease of use;
Time efficient;
Create an audit trail.

In an MCDA, you are comparing the utility of different options. Therefore, the application of MCDA is much more straightforward compared to other decision analysis tools such as decision trees. In an analysis based on decision trees, you must account for the subjective nature of utility. For example, we tend to use discounted cash flow in a decision tree, this discounting creates a bias – a preference – towards near time positive cash flows. The higher the discount rate, the higher the preference for near time positive cash flows becomes. Risk attitude is another factor that can create a biases. This opposed to MCDA where we simply order alternatives in terms of preference, i.e., utility.

Defining the problem

Patients may have multiple clinical trials in which they could participate. However, I advise you to seek advice from your doctor to create a list of trials for which you qualify.

A searchable list of clinical trials can be found at https://clinicaltrials.gov/.

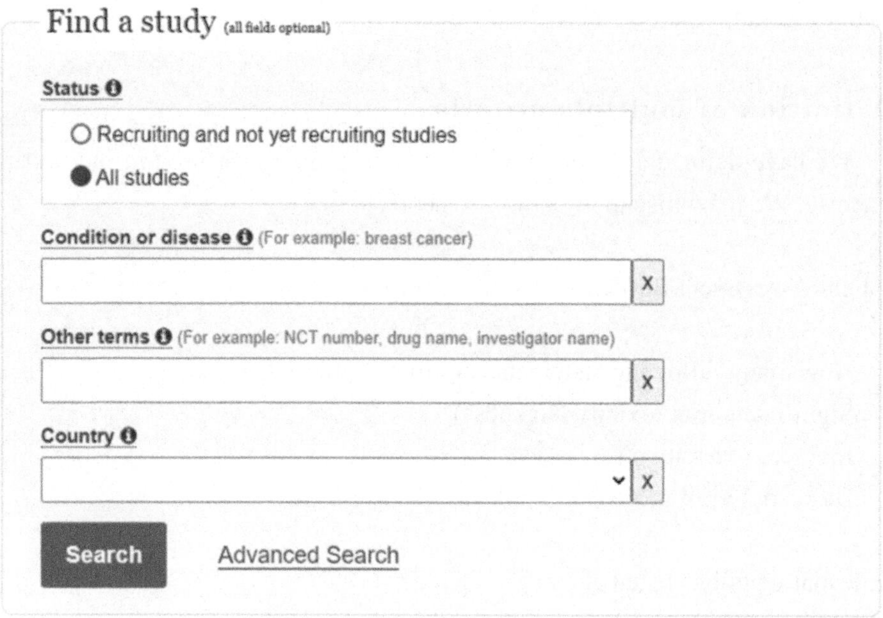

Find a study (all fields optional)

Status ❶

○ Recruiting and not yet recruiting studies

● All studies

Condition or disease ❶ (For example: breast cancer)

[   ] X

Other terms ❶ (For example: NCT number, drug name, investigator name)

[   ] X

Country ❶

[⌄] X

Search   Advanced Search

Figure 7.6. Screenshot from https://clinicaltrials.gov/, which allows doctors and patients to search for relevant clinical trials.

The website has extensive search options (Figure 7.6), and you can create a list of ongoing trials that are currently looking for patients, i.e., recruiting. All trials have eligibility criteria, i.e., the conditions that patients need to comply with. The eligibility criteria and the participating hospitals and doctors are also listed.

After you have created a list of the clinical trials that you both qualified for and are interested in participating in, you need to collect data on the characteristics of each of the trials on the list. The data are used in the scoring of the trials. MCDA is used to rank the clinical studies according to your preferences. These preferences are defined by your strategic objectives (see chapter *Values*). In this section, we refer to these fundamental objectives as criteria. Five criteria were defined: Patient Assessment Burden, Patient Visit Burden, Patient Logistical Burden[148], Clinical Phase, and Science. The data must show a degree of variability. In situations where a certain issue or criteria does

---

[148] The first three criteria are collectively referred to as "patient burden".

not differentiate between alternatives, simply remove the issue from the list. No matter how important the perceived value is.

Definition of multiple criteria

We have defined a series of attributes that can be measured in the scoring exercise. We maximise their combined score.

Patient Assessment Burden:

How many following statements are true (Table 7.1):
Significant drug toxicity (sickness);
Invasive assessments;
Blood draws of more than 3 ml.

How many options listed above are TRUE?

Score[149]	Answer[150]
3	0
2	1
1	2 or 3

Table 7.1. Patient Assessment Burden Score.

Patient Visit Burden:
Patient Visit Burden is determined by two factors:
Treatment duration (in days);
Number of annual tests (procedures per year per patient).

Patient Visit Burden Score is the product of these two factors[151]:
Patient Visit Burden Score

$$= \text{Treatment duration} * \text{Number of annual tests}$$

---

[149] This is the score of the Patient Assessment Burden that is aggregated with the other assessments made.

[150] Patient Assessment Burden should be an alternative listed in this column.

[151] Patient Visit Burden Score=Treatment duration*Number of annual tests=60*10=600.

Patient Logistical Burden:

Patient Logistical Burden is determined by three factors:

Number of visits (natural scale);

Travel time (in hours);

Travel cost (in pounds);

Length of any visit (in hours).

Patient Logistical Burden Score is the product of these four factors:

$$\text{Patient Visit Logistical Score}$$
$$= \text{Number of visits} * \text{Travel time} * \text{Travel cost}$$
$$* \text{Lenght of any visit}$$

Clinical Phase[152]:

Phase 1a or Phase 2a: Tests for safety, side effects, and optimal dose (Table 7.2);

Phase 2b: Test for efficacy (how well the drug works at the prescribed dose(s));

Phase 2/3: Test how well a new treatment works for a certain type of cancer and compare the new treatment with standard treatment. The latter is also referred to as the Standard of Care.

---

[152] Drug development for oncology drugs is slightly different from the traditional process of drug development. In Phase 2a oncology, patients are treated instead of healthy volunteers in traditional Phase 1. For rather obvious reasons, it is unethical to expose healthy individuals to toxic anti-cancer drugs. Phase 3 in the combined Phase 2/3 studies tended to be smaller than conventional standalone Phase 3 studies. Traditional drug development consists of three clinical trials: Phase 1 (safety testing in healthy volunteers), Phase 2 (how well does the drug work in patients), and Phase 3 (confirmative study to test whether the drug also works in a large group of patients).

What is the current clinical phase?

Score	Answer
3	Phase 2/3
2	Phase 2b
1	Phase 1a or Phase 2a

Table 7.2 Clinical phase.

Science:

Overall Survival is most probably unknown at the time of the study; therefore, it might not be considered of any relevance. However, overall survival is of most interest to the patient and is included mainly for illustrative purposes.

Overall Survival can be expressed using a natural scale in months.

The Scientific Rationale or *mechanism of action* relates to the way the drug works in the body. There is often a real benefit in changing the way a drug acts in the body, i.e., using a different *mechanism of action*. Therefore, if the user enters "Different" the logic enters a 2 into the formula shown below, and if the user enters "Same" a 1 is entered into the formula.

$$\text{Science} = \text{Overall Survival} * \text{Scientific Rational}$$

Normalisation across attributes

The following normalisation procedure can be applied to all criteria:

(1) Sum the raw weights for all attributes.
(2) Divide 1 by the sum of weights to obtain an adjustment factor.
(3) Multiply each raw weight by the adjustment factor.

This yields a set of weights that sum to 1.

For example, the Patient Assessment Burden:
(1) The five clinical studies received scores of 2, 2, 1, 0, and 1, respectively. The total equals 6.
(2) $\frac{1}{6} = 0.167$
(3) $0.167 * 2 = 0.333$; $0.167 * 1 = 0.167$; $0.167 * 0 = 0$

Clinical trial characteristics

Table 7.3 shows the scoring system used for the assessment of clinical trials.

	Clinical study A	Clinical study B	Clinical study C	Clinical study D	Clinical study E
Patient Assessment Burden:					
Significant drug toxicity (sickness)	No	Yes	Yes	Yes	Yes
Invasive assessments	No	No	Yes	Yes	Yes
Blood draws of more than 3 ml	No	No	No	Yes	No
Raw Score:	2	2	1	0	1
Score:	0.333	0.333	0.167	0	0.167
Patient Visit Burden:					
Treatment duration (in days)	10	20	30	12	12
Number of annual tests (procedures per year per patient)	5	3	1	10	10
Raw Score:	50	60	30	120	120
Score:	0.132	0.158	0.079	0.316	0.316
Patient Logistical Burden:					
Number of visits (natural scale)	22	11	5	5	5
Travel time (in hours)	1.5	1.5	1.5	1.5	1.5
Travel cost (in pounds)	120	120	120	120	120
Treatment cost (in pounds) Enter "1" if no personal contribution is required	1	1	1	1	1
Length of any visit (in hours)	8	8	10	10	6
Raw Score:	31680	15840	9000	9000	5400
Score:	0.447	0.223	0.127	0.127	0.076
Clinical Phase:					
Clinical phase	Phase 2/3	Phase 2b	Phase 1a or Phase 2a	Phase 1a or Phase 2a	Phase 2/3
Raw Score:	3	2	1	1	3
Score:	0.3	0.2	0.1	0.1	0.3
Science:					
Overall Survival (in months)	90	50	90	50	80

Scientific Rationale (Mechanism of action)	Same	Same	Different	Different	Different
Raw score:	90	50	180	100	160
Score:	0.155	0.086	0.31	0.172	0.276

Table 7.3. Scores of clinical trials.

Weighting of the criteria

Importance weights are used to express the relative importance of each criterion. The sum of these important weights should be 100%.

A normalisation procedure can be used to ensure that the sum of the weights is 100%. The procedure employed is as follows:

(1) Assign each attribute an integer from 0 to 10 to represent its raw weight;
(2) Sum the raw weights for all attributes;
(3) Divide 1 by the sum of weights to obtain an adjustment factor and;
(4) Multiply each raw weight by the adjustment factor.

This procedure yields a set of weights that sum to 1. Table 7.4 shows an example of importance weights.

Criteria	Raw weights	Weights
Patient Assessment Burden	2	18.2%
Patient Visit Burden	2	18.2%
Patient Logistical Burden	2	18.2%
Clinical Phase	4	36.4%
Science	1	9.1%
	Total: 11	
	Adjustment factor: 0.11	

Table 7.4. An example of the calculation of importance weights. Patient Assessment Burden = 18.2% = 2/0.11.

The highest weight was given to the *Clinical Phase*. In my judgement, the value of comparing clinical trials is largely determined by how far the project has progressed in its development. I gave the *Science* the lowest weight because we simply might not know what the Overall Survival is.

Multi-Criteria Decision Analysis results

Figure 7.7 shows an example of the output of the MCDA. Clinical trial A has the highest score, so it is the preferred option. Clinical trial A scores higher than Clinical trial E because it has a more favourable profile on the *Patient Assessment Burden* and the *Patient Logistical Burden* despite scoring lower on the *Patient Visit Burden* and *Science* criteria.

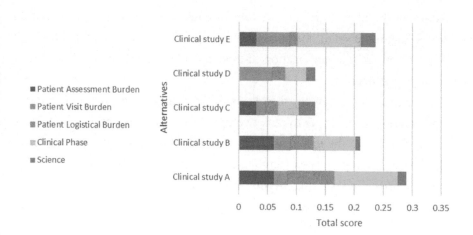

Figure 7.7. An example of scoring clinical trials using eight criteria in an application of Multi-Criteria Decision Analysis.

A digital copy of the Excel file used to create the plot above can be found in the repository of this book.

Swing weights

The application of *swing weights*[153] is generally considered to be the most correct and accurate method for deriving criterion weights.

One can apply the method using the algorithm shown below:

a) Assign a score of one to the alternative, in this case a trial, that best satisfies that criterion

b) Identify the alternative that least satisfies the criteria and use a choice listed in your judgement:

---

[153] Von Winterfeldt and Edwards, 1986.

- score 0 if the option is unacceptable (0 is the minimum value);
- score 0.5 if the option is very significantly worse than the best option;
- score 0.75 if the option is significantly worse than the best option;
- score 0.90 if the option is slightly worse than the best option.

c) Score the remaining options relative to the highest and lowest scores, now you have identified the top and the bottom alternatives.

Note that the algorithm must be run for each of the criteria. It is common practice to identify a set of objectives, the algorithm needs to be applied for each of those objectives. The application of this algorithm results in a ranked list of items for each objective.

This approach caters to the strength of humans in making relative judgements. It is much easier to rank two options on a relative basis than to rank the actual quantity of the difference. For example, it is easy for people to detect a temperature difference when stepping into another room but quantifying this temperature difference – quantifying the temperature difference in degrees Celsius – is a much harder task. Likewise, it is also easy to create an ordinal ranking of a series of alternatives.

Constructed scales

Many metrics lack a natural scale, and in those cases, one must resort to developing a constructed scale. We can use simple words to describe different states. Especially in situations with many alternatives, this approach simplifies the actual scoring process. In cases where there are many alternatives, it is difficult to hold all the values in your memory[154]. Table 7.5 lists the sets of constructed scales. You can see that the number of options available can vary among different criteria.

---

[154] Although this difficulty can be addressed by automatically re-ordering the items that have been scored.

Category	Overall survival (in months)	Treatment duration (in months)	Invasive assessment	Reputation of the sponsoring company
1	60 or more	Less than 2	No	Excellent
2	Between 24 (inclusive) and 60	Between 2 (inclusive) and 5	Yes	Average
3	Between 12 (inclusive) and 24	Between 4 (inclusive) and 8		Poor
4	Less than 12	8 or more		Unacceptable

Table 7.5. Scoring categories for different scales.

Two words of caution:

1) Using the constructed scale method of scoring can lead to a *compression of scale*. For example, an overall survival of 1 week is fundamentally different from an overall survival of 11 months. Despite this fact, both alternatives will receive an identical score. A potential solution is to redefine the answers or create additional options.

2) Scoring can introduce a bias as analysts make a judgement that a particular trial is of "average length" and consequently experts could preferentially select the middle option if this option represents the "average length" of a trial.

Decision Quality

[Difficulty: Green]

We make thousands of decisions every single day. The decisions we face relate to an almost infinite range of issues and levels of complexity. *Decision Quality* enables you to:

Judge the quality of your decisions as you make them;
Avoid the most common heuristic (rule-of-thumb) biases that undermine decision making;
Navigate today's uncertainty with confidence; and
Execute your decisions with greater buy-in and success.

Decision Quality is a framework that explicitly recognises six elements (Figure 7.8). The Decision Quality elements are often visualised as links in a chain symbolising that a decision is only as good as its weakest link, i.e., the decision element of the poorest quality. That is the place the decision maker should focus its effort.

The decision maker should structure his or her work around these six elements and check whether all Decision Quality elements have been explored at the time a decision is to be made.

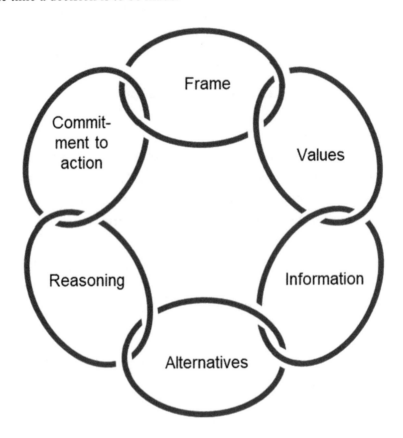

Figure 7.8. The six elements of decision quality. The diagram is shown as a chain because it symbolises the weakest link, the weakest link on which you must focus your effort.

Decision Quality as an overarching process

One can create a process around decision analysis. The structure of the process and the focus questions are shown in Figure 7.9. Decision analysis can be an iterative process where several cycles might be needed to focus on the critical aspect of a decision. Also, note that the definition of the *appropriate frame* and *clear values* is not revisited when iterating through the process.

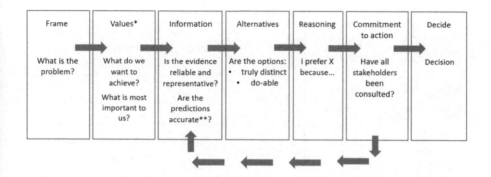

Figure 7.9. Decision analysis framework. *Values are discussed in the previous chapter, **Information can be either firmly established (the first question listed) or extrapolated/estimated (the second question listed).

There are also various tools that can be integrated into decision analysis. The tools are indicated in the decision analysis process chart (Figure 7.10).

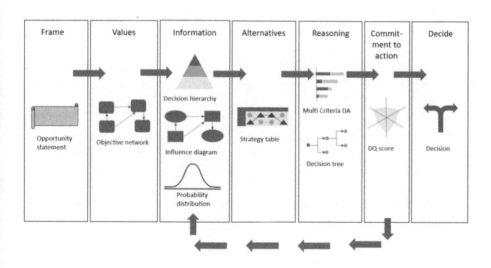

Figure 7.10. Decision analysis toolkit.

It rarely happens that all decision analysis tools are required. Most often, two to four tools are sufficient to obtain the insight needed to be confident in a decision. Table 7.6 lists all the decision analysis tools. In the final column, the purpose of each tool is summarised.

Tool Symbol/name		Decision quality element	Purpose
	Opportunity statement	Frame	An opportunity statement is a short description of the problem you are trying to solve.
	Objective network	Value	What do you truly care about?
	Decision hierarchy	Information	What are the decisions we should focus on?
	Influence diagram	Information	An influence diagram visualises issues and their relationships
	Probability distribution	Information	A probability distribution is a description of outcomes that are more likely than others.
	Strategy table	Alternatives	A strategy table can be used to develop distinct alternatives.
	Multi Criteria Decision Analysis	Reasoning	Multi Criteria Decision Analysis is used to rank alternatives.
	Decision tree	Reasoning	Decision tree is used to define logic using uncertainties and future decisions.
	Decision Quality	Commitment to action	Decision quality provides guidance on how your decision can be improved.

Table 7.6. An overview of the decision analysis tool described in this book.

Concluding remarks: Decision analysis

Decision analysis is a collection of methods that can help to create a structure around a decision and provide guidance on how one could improve the decision, i.e., increase the likelihood of ending up in a desirable situation. Decision analysis enables people to analyse a situation, communicate their value system and develop insight. Once these insights have been developed, the optimal choice should be obvious.

In the next two chapters, *Willingness to Pay* and *Innumeracy* are of particular interest to patients who are facing a severe illness. In Willingness to Pay, an attempt is made to quantify the value of life. Innumeracy is an introduction to statistics, but the examples discussed are mainly medical in nature. The third chapter following this chapter, *Human judgement,* describes how to create reasonable judgements.

Willingness to Pay

'Man only likes to count his troubles; he doesn't calculate his happiness.'

Fyodor Dostoevsky in *Notes from Underground, White Nights, The Dream of a Ridiculous Man, and Selections from The House of the Dead.*

'The surgeon lifts the chopped-out pear high into the air, whilst everyone else in the operating theatre drops to their knees in awe.'

Adam Blain in *Pear Shaped*

Abstract Willingness to Pay

Willingness to Pay is the amount of money a healthcare provider is willing to pay per year for a treatment of a medical condition. The NHS has been using £20k to £30k since 1999[155]. An often-quoted value for the US is $50k[156]. This latter number originates from the 1980s and represents the annual cost of a dialysis patient suffering from kidney failure. After correction for inflation, this number increases to $130k in nominal 2023 dollars. A recent study quoted a wide range of values for Willingness to Pay from $12k to $590k[157].

The average direct per-patient medical cost for brain tumours is £13k[158]. This is higher than that for breast, lung, or prostate cancer. Of course, this monetary amount varies dramatically depending on the patient. For those with a higher-grade malignant tumour, the direct medical cost for a year can be as high as £180k[159].

---

[155] For the relevant reference, the reader is directed to the main text in the chapter.

[156] Grosse, 2008

[157] Yong et al., 2022.

[158] https://www.braintumourresearch.org/

[159] https://www.braintumourresearch.org/

I was told by the medical team prior to the operation that they could not identify the type of tumour that was growing in my brain. Therefore, the medical team could not tell whether the cost was closer to £13k or closer to £180k.

In my judgement in mid-June 2022, I will have a Quality of Life of 100% until the brain tumour starts growing again. Therefore, my life is worth £9k per month as long as the tumour is not reducing my Quality of Life. Once it starts growing, I believe that I will have six months of linear decline until death. This profile of Quality of Life has an expected value of around £120k. This value of £120k falls in range between £13k and £180k.

There is just one problem with this calculation; most of the assumptions are poorly constrained and virtually unknowable: the discount rate, the development of Quality of Life over time, the length of the treatment, and the fact that as patients gets older, the Willingness to Pay is reduced. The uncertainty around the input values, and the fact that the value of a Quality Adjusted Life Years is also poorly constrained, makes the entire approach effectively useless.

How much is a life worth?

[Difficulty: Blue]

Willingness to Pay is the amount of money a healthcare provider (e.g., a hospital) is willing to pay for a drug or operation. The NHS follows the advice provided by the National Institute for Health and Clinical Excellence (NICE). NICE has been using a cost-effective range of £20k to £30k ever since it was created in 1999[160]. One value that is also often quoted is $50k[161]. In 1980s, this was the monetary value spent on the annual cost of a dialysis patient suffering from kidney failure. Given that these numbers were estimated several decades ago, inflation alone would triple this nominal cost. The nominal value of $50k in 1985 equates to over $130k in 2023[162].

Over the past three decades, almost 600 interventions, including injury reductions, toxin control, and new drugs and surgical procedures, have indicated an extremely broad range of values. There were some interventions that saved more resources than they cost, while others were costing more than 10 billion

[160] McCabe et al., 2008; Gandjour, 2020.

[161] Grosse, 2008

[162] https://www.worlddata.info/america/usa/inflation-rates.php#:~:text=During%20the%20observation%20period%20from,year%20inflation%20rate%20was%207.1%25

dollars per life per year[163]. A 2022 paper by Yong et al. examined 54 health economic studies published after 2000 and reported that the quoted Willingness to Pay, for a human to live one additional year, ranged from $12k to $590k.

Despite this very large range of Willingness to Pay, there is one obvious way to determine the price for a new drug or operation. Price benchmarking could be used by comparing the effect of the novel drug with the effect of existing treatments. Following this approach, one could argue that if treatment A is deemed superior to treatment B, treatment A should fetch a higher price than treatment B. One could speculate that price differences might persist over time as a consequence of such approach to settling on a price for a particular treatment. There might certain diseases where the Willingness to Pay is simply higher than the average. If that is true, there most then also be situations where the Willingness to Pay is lower...

Willingness to Pay and brain cancer

[Difficulty: Green]

At £13k[164], the average direct per-patient medical cost for brain tumours is significantly higher than that for breast, lung or prostate cancer. Of course, this varies dramatically depending on the patient. For higher-grade malignant tumour cost can reach an enormous £180k. On a per-patient basis, brain tumours are the second most expensive condition overall (after neuromuscular disorders). The costs of treating the mental health aspects of brain tumours at approximately £150 per patient seem largely irrelevant in the bigger picture.

I am very grateful that the NHS settled this bill for me because it turned out that my tumour was a high-grade tumour.

Correction of the Quality of Life value

[Difficulty: Green]

What are the benefits associated with extending your life by 6 months? One consideration relates to your age. The younger you are, the higher the Willingness to Pay for a high Quality of Life (QoL). This is not just because the expected number of years of life remaining is greater for a young person than for an elderly person. This is also because we as a society, are willing to pay more

---

[163] Tengs et al., 1995.

[164] https://www.braintumourresearch.org/

for a young person than for an elderly person. One study estimated that Willingness to Pay for someone in his/her 40s is about 40% higher than that for someone in their 80s[165]. It becomes even more complicated if multiple time horizons need to be considered. How about a single month for 10-year-old versus 12 months for an 80-year-old?

Another issue with the QoL score is that it fails to acknowledge that some patients perceive their current QoL as worse than that of death. This indicates that not everyone would assign the lowest score on the QoL scale to "death."

Pain and QoL

Early morning, on the 14th of May 2022, during my steroid-induced awakenings, I felt fortunate. At this point in time, the brain tumour had not affected my Quality of Life, neither physically nor mentally. I was also thinking about my dad. Dad was likely to be awake at the same time because of the same steroid side effects. Dad was in much pain.

One year later, in June 2023, Dad is still in severe pain and has become bedridden. After a short shuffle across the living room, he must lie down to relieve himself from the worst of his back pain. My Dad is the living proof that the commonly heard comment 'there is no need for patients to be in pain' is a falsehood – this statement is simply not true. My Dad has been suffering from chronic pain for decades. His pain has kept him awake for countless nights.

I read a BBC article stating that one in four people are living with chronic pain. BBC reported 'Chronic pain, defined as pain that lasts longer than three months, can drastically change people's lives. It can be caused by a physical problem, such as a slipped disc, but can also occur with no clear cause, known as primary pain. It destroys careers, breaks up relationships, steals independence and denies people the futures they had imagined.'

Atul Gawande is an oncologist who wrote about the suffering of his dying father[166] and his terminally ill patients in his emotional book *Being Mortal*: 'Pain often stands in the way – prevents – surviving. Human survival requires the

---

[165] Brey and Pinto Prades, 2017.

[166] Atul describes how his father became progressively more disabled because of spinal cord cancer and how, at least during the early stages of his disease, he continued his work as a surgeon despite increasing discomfort in his hands.

ability to breath, drink, urinate, excrete, stay warm, and sleep. These needs are the biological components of human survival[167].'

Pain is a very subjective phenomenon. However, no matter how subjective pain is, it will always have a negative impact on the patient's Quality of Life.

Incremental Cost Effectiveness Ratio

[Difficulty: Black]

The term "cost effectiveness" is seldom absent from a discussion of money and health care, but it has often been presented with the erroneous premise that saving money should be the sole objective[168]. The objective should instead be to maximise the benefits given budgetary constraints. A commonly used metric is the incremental cost effectiveness ratio (ICER)[169] given by:

$$ICER = \frac{Cost\ of\ X - Cost\ of\ Y}{Benefit\ of\ X - Benefit\ of\ Y}$$

One problem with the way ICER is calculated is that you could end up with identical ICER values using different assumptions. The example shown in Table 8.1 illustrates how preferences change from one option to another. In this example, the benefits are kept constant and the differences in cost are also fixed. Hence, there is no difference in the ICER; both are equal to 1. However, there is a change of preference in ICER_proposed.

	Cost	Benefit	ICER	ICER_proposed	
X1	20	4	$\frac{20-18}{4-2}=1$	$\frac{20}{4}<\frac{18}{2}$	Y is preferred
Y1	18	2			
X2	3	4	$\frac{3-1}{4-2}=1$	$\frac{3}{4}>\frac{1}{2}$	X is preferred
Y2	1	2			

Table 8.1. Comparison of the two treatments and their cost and benefits.

Why are we still using the ICER method? It baffles me to be honest...

---

[167] Maslow, 1943.

[168] Doublet et al., 1986.

[169] ICER is the equivalent of the inverse of Return On Investment (ROI).

To use ICER, we need a method to define the *benefit*. Quality Adjusted Life Years might seem like an obvious choice, but is it?

Quality of Life and Quality Adjusted Life Years

[Difficulty: Black]

Quality of Life (QoL) can be scored from 0 to 1, where 0 signifies death and 1 indicates that the individual feels completely healthy. An example of how QoL can change is illustrated in Figure 8.1 by the blue line, in which QoL remains constant at 1 for the first seven years, drops to 0.4 in the seventh year, and remains constant for the next five years. In contrast, the grey line is a constant 0.9 for the full 12 years. Looking at Figure 8.1 it should be obvious that the grey line is preferred over the blue line, the question is how many Quality Adjusted Life Years (QALY) would one gain if you could move from the blue line to the grey line?

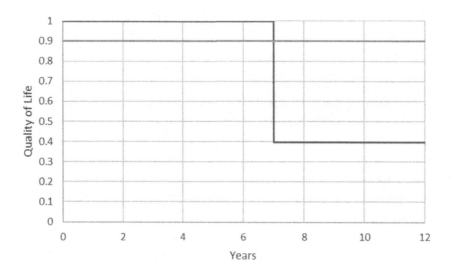

Figure 8.1. Two Quality of Life scenarios.

The QALY benefit can be calculated using the following formula:

$$QALY = 7 * (0.9 - 1) + 5 * (0.9 - 0.4) = -0.7 + 2.5 = 1.8$$

A QALY is the total number of life years gained by a certain treatment. The example described above illustrates how QALYs can be calculated in scenarios where the QoL is less than 100% but persists over many years.

Monetary value of human life

[Difficulty: Black]

When patients are subjected to a treatment that makes them very sick for a significant part of their short remaining life, how do you balance patient burden against a small extension of their life?

The monetary value of a year's life is $130k[170] or £108. The monetary value of a month is then given by:

$$Value\ of\ single\ month\ of\ life = L = \frac{108}{12} = £9k\ per\ month$$

Therefore, having a QoL of 100% is worth £9k per month.

Economists address risk[171] by reducing a monetary amount that is to be paid out at some time in the future by a certain percentage. The higher the degree of

---

[170] Based on the annual nominal cost of a dialysis patient in 1985, which has been inflated to determine the real cost in 2023.

[171] Economists make a distinction between market risk and private risk. Market risk reflects the mood of the market. In a bull market, share prices are expected to increase. The reverse happens in a bear market when the temperament of the market is depressed and share prices are expected to decrease. Market risk affects the price of all shares being traded and cannot be eliminated.

In contrast, private risk affects the shares of a single company. For example, the failure of a trial sponsored by a pharmaceutical company will lower its share price. However, such a failure should not affect the share prices of companies in other industries such as automotive, energy, or electronics. However, the failure of a drug trial might affect the share prices of other pharmaceutical companies. A given drug is intended to work with a particular mechanism in the human body, and drugs that share this mechanism are considered to be from the same class. When the drug from a certain class fails, the impact of its failure is likely to negatively affect the share price of those competitors that are developing drugs in that same class. An investor can mitigate this private risk by owning shares in a diverse portfolio of companies.

Modelling the impact of private risk is relatively straightforward. One applies a fixed percentage reduction to the value of the project, i.e., the entire future cash flow will be

risk, the higher the risk penalty you pay. This risk penalty is referred to as the discount rate, or d. The penalty function is cumulative. Assume there is an annual monetary amount of £100 to be realised over the next three years, and also assume a discount rate of 10%. The £100 realised in the first year will remain at £100, the £100 realised in the second year will be reduced to £90 $\left(\frac{100}{(1+0.1)} = 90\right)$ and finally the £100 realised in the third year will be reduced to £83 $\left(\frac{100}{(1+0.1)^2} = 83\right)$. The total value is the sum of all discounted values. This total is referred to as the Net Present Value. The Net Present Value of this three year long project is equal to £100 + £90 + £83 = £273.

I do not see any reason why one could not make financial assessments of treatment regimens involving chronic diseases.

For a patient who receives a 20-year treatment, under the assumption that the patient has a QoL of 100% during the entire duration of the treatment, the Net Present Value is given by:

$$Net\ Present\ Value = \sum_{0}^{t=20} \frac{C_t}{(1+d)^t}$$

where C_t is £9k given that the QoL is 100%[172],

d is the discount rate,

and t is the period.

---

reduced by the same percentage. The percentage chosen is commonly referred to as the Chance of Success. The percentage applied is a number that is based on a judgment, so we are back to the world of psychology!

[172] If the QoL is let's say 50% the C_t will proportionally be reduced, i.e., one halves the Net Present Value.

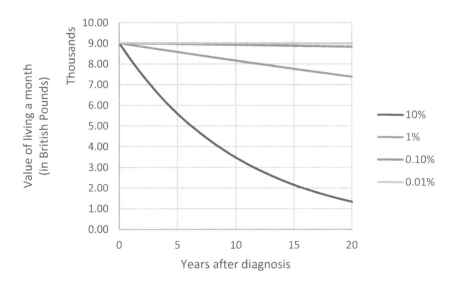

Figure 8.2. Quality of Life development as a function of the chosen discount rate.

The Net Present Value drops off very quickly at an annual discount rate of 10%, whereas under the assumption that the annual discount rate is 0.01%, there is virtually no reduction over the 20-year period (Figure 8.2).

The impact of the discount rate is also obvious in the comparison of the value created by treating patients with a chronic disease. Table 8.2 shows that under the assumption of an annual discount rate of 10%, the value created is £86k, whereas under the assumption of an annual discount rate of 0.01%, the value created is £189k.

Annual discount rate	Value of life (in £'000)
10%	86
1%	172
0.10%	188
0.01%	189

Table 8.2. The value of a 20-year treatment given that QoL is 100%.

The longer the expected life remaining, the more pronounced is the effect of the discount factor. In my case, where the median survival was set at 16 months at the time of diagnosis, discounting the value of a month's life has little impact.

However, many other chronic diseases take their course over many decades, in which case discounting will have a significant impact on the total value of life.

It is also very clear from the numbers we calculated that the result is very sensitive to the assumptions we enter into the formula[173]. Depending on the assumptions entered, one calculates values that are vastly different. Most of the assumptions are poorly constrained and virtually unknowable; the discount rate, the development of QoL over time, the length of the treatment, and the fact that as patients get older, the willingness to pay is reduced. The uncertainty around the input values, combined with the fact that the value of a QALY is also poorly constrained, makes the entire approach effectively useless…

In principle, theoretically, we can calculate whether the benefits of the removal of the brain tumour outweigh the cost. In other words, whether the NHS made a good investment by operating a patient like me.

I suspect that once the tumour starts growing, it cannot be restrained. I suspect that, over a period of six months, QoL will drop from 100% to 0%. In the absence of any detailed knowledge, I assumed that the drop would occur linearly. The start of the decline in my QoL starts in the period 11 (Table 8.3).

The value of a patient with glioblastoma can be calculated using the formula below:

$$Net\ Present\ Value = \sum_{t=0}^{10} \frac{L_t * Q_t}{(1+d)^t} + \sum_{t=11}^{16} \frac{1-(t-t_{10})}{t_{17}-t_{10}} * \frac{L_t * Q_t}{(1+d)^t}$$

where L represents Monetary value of single month of life,
where Q represents Quality of Life,
t represents time in months,

$Multiplier = 1$ if $t \leq 10, \frac{1-(t-t_{10})}{t_{17}-t_{10}}$ if $t > 10$ and
d represents the discount rate.

The calculated results are shown in Table 8.3. The different totals indicate the impact of various discount rates.

----

[173] Several years ago, I tried to determine the discount rate for the firm I was working for and ran into the same problem…

Month	Multiplier	Annual discount rate:			
		0.1	0.01	0.001	0.0001
0	1	£9,000	£9,000	£9,000	£9,000
1	1	£8,925	£8,993	£8,999	£9,000
2	1	£8,851	£8,985	£8,999	£9,000
3	1	£8,778	£8,978	£8,998	£9,000
4	1	£8,705	£8,970	£8,997	£9,000
5	1	£8,633	£8,963	£8,996	£9,000
6	1	£8,561	£8,955	£8,996	£9,000
7	1	£8,490	£8,948	£8,995	£8,999
8	1	£8,420	£8,940	£8,994	£8,999
9	1	£8,350	£8,933	£8,993	£8,999
10	1	£8,280	£8,925	£8,993	£8,999
11	0.86	£7,062	£7,669	£7,733	£7,739
12	0.71	£5,782	£6,326	£6,384	£6,389
13	0.57	£4,603	£5,075	£5,124	£5,129
14	0.43	£3,444	£3,825	£3,865	£3,870
15	0.29	£2,303	£2,578	£2,607	£2,610
16	0.14	£1,103	£1,243	£1,258	£1,260
17	0.00	£0	£0	£0	£0
Life's value		£119,290	£125,306	£125,931	£125,993

Table 8.3. Valuation results for different discount rates.

The operation is estimated to cost between £13k and £180k[174]. I was told by the medical team prior to the operation that they could not identify the tumour growing in my brain. Therefore, the medical team could not tell whether the cost was closer to £13k or closer to £180k. Given that my prognosis is so poor, the impact of the discount rate is more or less irrelevant. The value of the life of a patient like me, £120k, falls in the range – which is a relief – or a coincidence – or both[175].

---

[174] https://braintumourresearch.org/blogs/research-campaigning-news/the-high-price-of-brain-tumours

[175] I did not consider my second operation. That would really muddle the water…and by the way; I did survive the period I considered in this analysis!

Concluding remarks: Willingness to Pay

Willingness to Pay is a monetary number that is impossible to calculate with a degree of precision that is required. As most of the assumptions are poorly constraint, virtually unknowable or very subjective, the determination of the Willingness to Pay remains elusive. Despite an impressive arsenal of methods and jargon, a reliable calculation of Willingness to Pay has yet to be identified.

I fully agree with Atul Gawande, who in *Being Mortal* states, 'Terminal cancer patients wouldn't pay £64,000 for drugs, and end-stage heart failure patients wouldn't pay £40,000 for defibrillation offering at best a few months' survival. However, this argument ignores an important factor: the people who for these treatments aren't thinking of a few added months. They're thinking about years of additional life. They're thinking they're getting at least that lottery ticket's chance that their disease might not be a problem anymore.'

Maybe, just maybe, the healthcare providers and physicians do not want to know. Maybe Willingness to Pay is all smoke and mirrors…

After this sobering finding, the message of the following chapter, *Innumeracy*, is equally depressing[176]. The next chapter will demonstrate how our poor grasp of the underlying mathematical concepts prevents us from truly improving our decision-making practises. However, explanations are offered on the most common concepts used to analyse the data collected during clinical trials.

---

[176] For those readers who cannot cope with all the negativity I recommend reading Part 4 of this book!

Innumeracy

'Getting too deeply into statistics is like trying to quench a thirst with salty water.'

Paul Kalanithi in *When Breath Becomes Air*

'At the end you will still be confused but you will be confused about different things.'

Steve Begg in a discussion about Bayes' rule

Abstract Innumeracy

The lack of basic knowledge of mathematics is the main reason why mankind is unable to improve the quality of their decisions. As more and more data are used in our decision making, we need to ensure that all of us have at least a basic understanding of statistics.

The numbers created by mathematics and statistics, in particular, summarise and characterise the real world. These numbers create insight and aid communication of the complexity of the environment we all inhabit. Statistics utilise probability distributions to describe this environment. A probability distribution, in its most basic form, is nothing more than an opinion on which scenario is the most likely to occur.

Our poor grasp of statistics makes us vulnerable to manipulation. Reporting metrics that make a treatment look more favourable than the data implies. Many doctors simply do not understand basic statistics and consequently fail to explain survival data to their patients. The prospects for a patient to gain a sufficient understanding of his/her illness are slim when the patient is not educated in statistics and diseases.

Even basic percentages, which are one of the most natural and least confusing of all the measures of treatment effect in clinical trials, are not understood by many patients and doctors.

Bayes' rule is introduced as a rigorous method to update one's belief in light of new data that becomes available over time.

Once you have finished reading this chapter, you should have sufficient statistical knowledge to have an educated conversation with your doctor.

Visit to the Waterstones in Oban

[Difficulty: Blue]

In April 2022, I visited Oban on the Scottish west coast. I was joined by my family and my mother-in-law. After buying some local scallops and langoustine (large shrimp) on the ferry front, I made my way to the Waterstones bookstore.

I have visited this shop many times over the past decades. I walked past sections of local interest, cooking, and history on my way to my favourite section: Popular Science. This section of books had been moved from where it was the last time, I visited the store. I looked around and ultimately found it. I was somewhat disappointed that the store decided not only to move the section but also to reduce it to a single unit about a metre wide with six or seven shelves. Familiar themes to the "popular scientist" included earth sciences, astronomy, and biology. I was drawn to the shelf labelled *mathematics*, where I found about six books about statistics and picked up a copy of *Outliers* by Malcolm Gladwell.

This book, I knew, would hold the key for a better understanding the world. Despite all the recent hype around machine learning and AI in popular films and series, prominent press releases on massive investment by data-hungry social media companies, and promises to revolutionise healthcare, people simply do not know how to deal with data, numbers, or statistics.

I estimated that only 2.9%[177] of the Oban Waterstones Popular Science section was allocated to popular statistics. The Popular Science section itself probably accounts for less than 2.5% of the total shelf space. This leaves 0.07%[178] of the total number of books at Waterstones to teach the general public about popular statistics.

---

[177] 6.5 statistical books / (6.5 shelves * 35 books per shelf) = 2.9%.

[178] 2.9% * 2.5% = 0.07%. The approach described above was inspired by Enrico Fermi, who estimated the number of piano tuners working in Chicago by breaking down the assessment into chunks for which he could use reliable estimates (e.g., the total population living in Chicago).

I also realise that only a small proportion of the people walking up and down the Oban harbour front will end up inside the Waterstones bookstore. In addition to fact that few books on statistics are available in Waterstones, the customers inside the store are not a representative sample of the general public. Most of the general public is relatively innumerate.

Statistical ignorance is rife.

Many people are wilfully innumerate. These people wear a badge of honour – 'I don't do maths!' This is a very serious matter. Let me quote John Allen Paulos, who wrote in his book, *Innumeracy*[179], the following:

'Though innumeracy may seem to be removed from people's real problems and concerns – money, sex, family, friends – it affects them (and all of us) directly and in many ways. If you walk down the main street of a resort town on a summer night, for example, and see happy people holding hands, eating ice-cream cones, laughing, etc., it is easy to think that other people are happier, more loving, more productive than you are and so become unnecessarily miserable. Yet it is precisely on such occasions that people display their good attributes, whereas they tend to hide and become "invisible" when they are depressed[180]. We should all remember that our impression of others is usually filtered in this way and that our sampling of people and their moods is not random. It's beneficial to occasionally wonder what percentage of people you encounter who suffer from this or that disease or inadequacy.'

In another section, Paulos talks about *Math Anxiety*:

'They're afraid [of mathematics]. They've been intimidated by officious and sometimes sexist teachers and others who may themselves suffer from math anxiety… They feel that there are mathematical minds and nonmathematical minds and that the former always come up with answers instantaneously whereas the latter are helpless and hopeless.'

---

[179] Paulos also wrote 'mathematics is too important to be left to mathematicians.' I am a Dutch geologist writing a textbook in English about decision analysis, statistics, and philosophy. I cannot think of anyone else who would be more qualified for writing this book than me!

[180] Paulos wrote this text in 1988, several decades before the advent of social media. In 2023 the likes of Instagram©, TikTok©, Facebook© and LinkedIn©, must have made the situation much worse compared to the situation described by Paulos. The online profile of a person is an idealised image that bears little resemblance to the actual person.

Innumeracy, the lack of basic knowledge of mathematics, is one of the hardest challenges that mankind faces. We would be able to make considerable progress in decision making, i.e., improve the quality of decisions, if we were able to discuss the implications of statistics. We use increasingly more data in our decision-making, but to reap the benefits from this deluge of data, we need to ensure that all of us have at least a basic understanding of statistics. I am acutely aware that many people, including doctors, struggle with this very topic.

Probability of a shared birthday

[Difficulty: Blue]

In our family, we have many people who celebrate their birthdays in the summer. Especially on my wife's side of the family. We tend to organise a single celebration for all birthdays that fall in the months of July and August. In fact, I can tell you that the number of birthdays in the summer months is much larger than the combined number of birthdays of the remainder of the year. But are birthdays truly more common in summer than in winter? Or is this an example where a pattern has arisen by chance and therefore is simply wrong? How about birthdays shared with famous people[181]?

One way to address this conundrum is to investigate the *birthday paradox*. The birthday paradox revolves around a simple question:

How many people does it take to be more than 50% certain that two people will share their birthday?

Answer:

23 people

Why does 23 seem like such a counterintuitive low answer?

People tend to think of their birthday and determine the probability that someone will have their birthday on the same date. However, the actual problem, as stated above, asks about any two individuals sharing their birthday. This means that you must compare all possible pairs of individuals. The source of confusion is related to the sheer number of possible combinations (Figure 9.1)[182]. The number of possible pairs increases much more rapidly than one would intuitively expect. Hence, the probabilities rise much more quickly than one initially believes.

---

[181] I share my birthday with Metallica rock singer James Hetfield.

[182] https://statisticsbyjim.com/fun/birthday-problem/

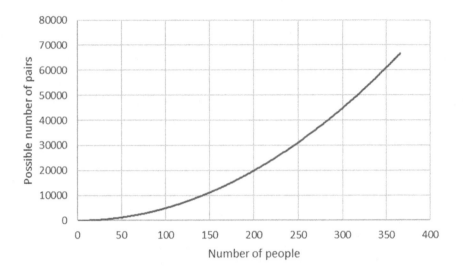

Figure 9.1. Possible number of pairs as a function of the number of people.

The logic behind the mathematics goes as follows: given that there are 23 individuals, the first person can be paired up with 22 individuals. The second person has already been paired up with the first person, so there are only 21 individuals left to make a new pair. The third person then has 20 potential partners, the fourth person has 19, and so on. If you add all possible combinations (22 + 21 + 20 + 19 + ... +1) it turns out that there are 253 combinations[183]. Consequently, each group of 23 people involved 253 combinations, and each of the 253 pairs could have a matched birthday.

Let's do the mathematics:

$$P(Shared\ birthday) = \left(\frac{Days\ in\ a\ year - 1}{Days\ in\ a\ year}\right)^{Number\ of\ possible\ pairs}$$

Or:

$$P(Shared\ birthday) = \left(\frac{365 - 1}{365}\right)^{253} = 0.4995 = 50\%$$

---

[183] The number of pairs of N people is equal to $(N * (N - 1))/2$.

A basic spreadsheet can be developed that tracks the probability of a shared birthday as a function of the number of people. The spreadsheet enables us to determine that the probability of a shared birthday is indeed around 50% for 23 individuals (Figure 9.2). The probability keeps going up – for 50 people, the probability is 97.0%; for 75 people, the probability is 99.97% – until the probability reaches a full 100%. This happens when the number of people reaches 366.

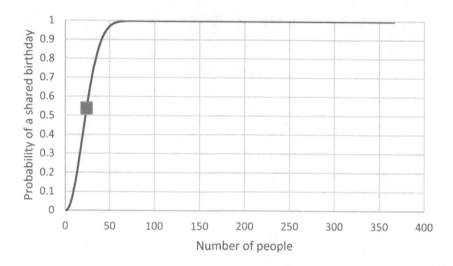

Figure 9.2. Probability of a shared birthday as a function of the number of people. The red symbol indicates 23 individuals and its probability of 50%.

An alternative solution to the birthday paradox

[Difficulty: Red]

What is the probability that two people share the same birthday[184]? The first person can be born on any day of the year, which means that the probability is $365/365 = 1$. The second person must be born on the same day as the first, and there is a 1/365 chance of that happening.

These two events should occur at the same time, so the probability is:

---

[184] The solution has been provided on the following webpage: https://www.cantorsparadise.com/ what-is-the-birthday-paradox-e72cc15832e1.

$$p(B) = \frac{365}{365} \times \frac{1}{365} = 0.0027 = 0.27\%$$

This low probability is in line with our expectations.

In practice it is much easier to determine the probability that a pair does not share the same birthday. This probability is denoted by $p'(B)$. To calculate the probability $p(b)$ based on $p'(B)$ we need to apply the following formula:

$$p(B) = 1 - p'(B) = 1 - \left(\frac{365}{365} \times \frac{364}{365}\right) = 0.27\%$$

For three people, this formula can be extended to:

$$p(B) = 1 - \left(\frac{365}{365} \times \frac{364}{365} \times \frac{363}{365}\right) = 0.83\%$$

Once the number of people is increased to 23, the calculation yields the following result[185]:

$$p(B) = 1 - \left(\frac{365}{365} \times \frac{364}{365} \times ... \times \frac{343}{365}\right) = 50.7\%$$

If the number of people is 23 or higher, one ends up with a probability that exceeds 50%.

What is a probability?

[Difficulty: Red]

I searched the web for a definition of "probability." This is one of them: 'A probability is a number that reflects the chance or likelihood that a particular event will occur. Probabilities can be expressed as proportions ranging from 0 to 1 or as percentages ranging from 0% to 100%.'[186]

---

[185] This formula can be rewritten as $p(B) = 1 - \left(\left(\frac{1}{365}\right)^{23} \times 365 \times 364 \times ... \times 343\right) = 50.7\%$.

[186] https://sphweb.bumc.bu.edu/otlt/mph-modules/bs/bs704_probability/BS704_Probability3.html

This definition reflects the fact that statistics has been dominated by thought experiments of flipping coins, throwing dice, drawing balls from a bag, and picking random cards from a deck. These experiments involve a well-defined set of outcomes, each of which have a known probability. This branch of statistics is referred to as *frequentist statistics*. Frequentist statistical problems are based on the premise that all outcomes are known and that each outcome has a known probability. Unfortunately, the problems we are typically dealing with are different. Bruno de Finetti famously stated: 'Probability does not exist'[187]. We simply do not know whether a coin is fair, whether a die is unweighted, how the proportion of red balls in a bag might change over time, or whether the cards are drawn from a standard deck.

In this type of problem, the probabilities are in themselves uncertain[188]. In addition, the number of outcomes might well be uncertain. This branch of statistics is referred to as *Bayesian statistics*. Bayesian statistics is one of the key pillars of decision analysis. In the late 1950s, at Harvard, Schlaifer and Raiffa began tackling business problems that were left unsolved by traditional, frequentist statisticians[189].

Bayesian statisticians consider probabilities as merely an aid to systematically quantify our beliefs about uncertainty. The rules of probability allow us to logically reason under uncertainty.

Bayesian statisticians would argue that there is no right or wrong probability assessments. If the assessment is a true reflection of the knowledge that is available to the expert, the assessment is valid. The assessment reflects your state of knowledge. The probability distribution is simply a quantification of that knowledge[190].

During a news briefing in 2002, Donald Rumsfeld stated:

---

[187] Nua, 2001.

[188] Gerd Gigerenzer distinguishes between "risk" and "uncertainty". "Risk" deals with problems with known outcomes, where each outcome has a well-defined probability. "Uncertainty" deals with problems in which the probability itself is unknown, also the number of outcomes is unknown.

[189] From scratch, they invented "tree flipping", conjugate priors, and started working on structured elicitation processes.

[190] Probability is a hotly debated topic among philosophers. The reader is referred to Suárez, 2021.

'…because as we know, there are known knowns; there are things we know we know. We also know that there are known unknowns; that is to say, we know that there are some things we do not know. But there are also unknown unknowns – the ones we don't know we don't know…'[191]

This lack of knowledge may appear intimidating. We simply do not know how many days, weeks, months, or years we have left to live. The cause of death for most of us is also unknown. Cancer, infection, cardiovascular disease, diabetes, accidents, pneumonia, and stroke are just a few of the causes.

Hans Rosling stated in his book *Factfulness*,[192] 'The world cannot be understood without numbers. And it cannot be understood by numbers alone.'

Updating a belief

[Difficulty: Red]

Upon accepting that a probability is no more than a belief, it is a small step to ascertain that upon learning something about a situation, one should update the probabilities. Bayes' rule should be used to update probabilities when new information becomes available.

The view without new information is referred to as a prior. The likelihood function is defined by the new information, and the posterior is the prior updated by the new information. In a Bayesian framework, all probabilities are defined as uncertain variables. This uncertain variable can be updated using Bayes' rule in a rigorous statistical fashion.

Bayes' rule can be illustrated by a basic example using a die. This example also clearly illustrates that probability is indeed a belief. What is the probability that the die you have just rolled has a *five* on top? Well, a cubic die has six sides, and a *five* is one of these six possibilities, so $1/6$. In a second experiment we pick up the dice, roll them again and cover the dice with a sheet of paper. We are very careful not to touch the die, i.e., the outcome is not changed after the roll. There is a little hole that shows the centre of the face of the die (Figure 9.3).

---

[191] Donald Rumsfeld gave a news briefing on February 12, 2002, about the lack of evidence linking the government of Iraq with the supply of weapons of mass destruction to terrorist groups. https://en.wikipedia.org/wiki/There_are_unknown_unknowns#cite_note-defense.gov-transcript-1.

[192] Rosling, 2018.

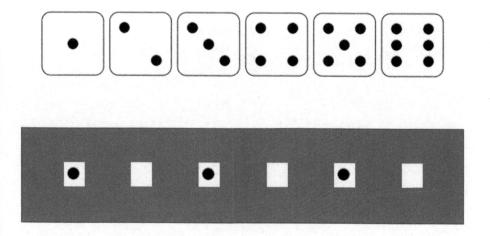

Figure 9.3. Uncertainty is a state of knowledge. The probability of throwing a *five* is ¹/₆. However, if we know whether a *dot* is in the middle of the die, we update our uncertainty to ¹/₃.

Guess what, there is a *dot*! With this new information available to inform your judgement, you are asked again: what is the probability that we have a *five*? Well, there are six possibilities, and three of those have a dot in the middle: *one*, *three*, and *five* (Figure 9.3). Because of this new information, we must revise our probabilities.

To apply Bayes' rule, we must role the die many times (the reader is referred to the following section for details). Let us say we role the die 6,000 times. From the 6,000 die throws, we expect 1,000 *fives* and 5,000 non-*fives*. All the 1,000 fives have a dot. For the non-fives, 2,000 have a dot while the remaining 3,000 have no dot. Now we can do the sums; $1,000 / (1,000 + 2,000) = ¹/₃$. Using *natural frequencies*, we can determine that the posterior probability is ¹/₃ (Figure 9.4).

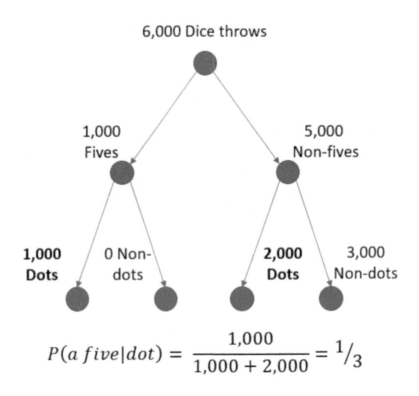

$$P(a\ five|dot) = \frac{1{,}000}{1{,}000 + 2{,}000} = \frac{1}{3}$$

Figure 9.4. Bayes' rule was applied to update our belief on throwing a *five*.
Note that even though no one touched the die, our probability assessment of a *five* has increased from $\frac{1}{6}$ to $\frac{1}{3}$.

Probability reflects the information in your head. Uncertainty is a function of the information available to you. Therefore, two people can make different assessments, yet both can be correct, provided that the assessments were based on all information available to them. Think about a new treatment for lung cancer. If you were to ask a board member of a pharmaceutical company about the likelihood of the treatment being successful, they will give you an answer based on historical data from past clinical trials. If you ask the same question to a member of the team involved in the development of that particular treatment, you get a different number. Why? Because the team member has more data available that is specific to the project. The project team has more project-specific knowledge than the board members. After the team has shared their knowledge with the board, the board member adjusts the likelihood to reflect this newly obtained knowledge.

Another example is an MRI scan image. The result of the MRI scan is uncertain to the patient before meeting the doctor. The doctor has studied the MRI scan prior to meeting the patient. Therefore, when the patient and the doctor meet, there is an asymmetry of information; the patient is still uncertain what is shown on the MRI scan, but the doctor already knows what is visible on the MRI scan.

Natural frequencies versus percentages

Gerd Gigerenzer argued in his book *Reckoning with Risk* for the use of natural frequencies rather than probabilities expressed as percentages. Therefore, rather than expressing the problem using percentages, Gigerenzer proposed using the actual number of patients and creating a probability tree to display the different groups. Natural frequencies facilitate inferences because they carry implicit information about base rates and reduce the number of computations required to determine the positive predictive value of a test.

Below is a recipe for developing a tree with natural frequencies[193]:
Step 1: Select a population and use the base rate to determine the number of people in the population with the disease.
Step 2: Take that result and apply the proportion of people with the disease and a positive test to determine the number of people with the disease.
Step 3: Take the remaining number of healthy people and use the test's false positive rate to determine how many people do not have the disease but still test positive.
Step 4: Compare the number obtained in step 2 with the sum of those obtained in steps 2 and 3 to determine how many people with a positive test have the disease.

Example of using natural frequencies:
Step 1: Figure 9.5 shows a tree that starts at the top with 10,000 individuals. Eighty of the ten thousand people have this rare disease.
Step 2: From those eighty people, 72 patients ended up with a positive result.

---

[193] Hoffrage et al., 2000.

Step 3: The remaining patients, 9920, were labelled as having "No disease". A positive test result was obtained by 694 patients. In this example, the number that is tested positive is dominated by false positives.

Step 4: There is only a 10% probability that a positive test result belongs to an individual with the disease (Figure 9.5).

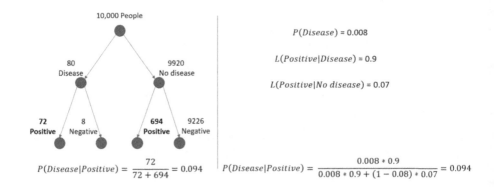

Figure 9.5. How natural frequencies facilitate Bayesian analysis.

The right panel from Figure 9.5 provides the traditional approach where the analyst enters percentages into Bayes's rule. Gigerenzer points out that using natural frequencies facilitates statistical reasoning, with minimal training or instruction.

Physics versus random

Flipping a coin is "physics" not "random". The outcome "heads" or "tails" of a coin flying through the air is determined by its initial conditions[194]. The outcome of the toss of a die is determined by the speed, spin, and height of the throw. Based on these initial conditions, Newton's Laws of physics enable us to calculate the outcome. Ignoring bias[195], landing on its side[196] or otherwise failing the get an outcome (e.g., sticking in the mud or the coin landing on a shoe), we can predict whether the coin will land "heads" or "tails."

---

[194] Diaconis et al., 2007.

[195] Typical flips show biases such as 0.495 or 0.503 (Diaconis, 2003).

[196] Apparently, the probability of this happening 1 in 6,000 tosses of an American nickel (Murray & Teare, 1993).

There is no randomness in a coin flip, nor is there randomness in the throw of a die. The outcome of rolling of a die or the flipping of a coin is controlled by the laws of physics. However, as anyone who has gambled can confirm, getting this initial condition consistently right is not a task for the fainthearted.

Methods of quantifying survival

[Difficulty: Red]

'You are not a statistic!'

The physician who found my brain tumour

When reading papers on clinical trials, several statistics are commonly reported. These statistics include:

Survival analysis and Hazard Ratio;
Mode, median, and mean;
Confidence interval;
Relative risk; and
Odds and Odds Ratio.

Survival analysis

The end of our lives

[Difficulty: Blue]

I realise that I am no different from the 8 billion fellow humans on this planet. We all will die one day. What makes my situation different is that I know the cause of my death, I have an idea of how the illness will affect the decline of my cognitive ability, and I have a decent view of the duration of my illness. I do realise that I am not the only one. There is an entire community out there. Or should I say communities? The list of chronic diseases is long: heart disease, cancer, COVID-19, unintentional injuries, stroke, chronic lower respiratory disease…the list goes on and on. Many diseases have many subcategories. Oncology, for example, is split into lung, breast, prostate, bladder…the list goes on and on. Brain cancer does not feature in the top 10 most common cancers.

However, if you are brave, or stupid, enough to type in "Brain cancer" in Google, you will end up with 0.66 seconds later with 1.150.000.000 hits.

The probability of any of you contracting one of these diseases within a given year is very small. In fact, even heart disease, which claims most lives in the US, is less than 0.2% on an annual basis. The probability of not having a heart failure is equal to 99.83%, i.e., just smaller than 1.

Although the probabilities are almost indistinguishable from 1 for all diseases, the point is that you are exposed to all of them. Even worse, every single year you must face all these risk factors once again. Table 9.1 shows the ten most common fatal diseases and the number of deaths per 100,000 US citizen[197]. As you can see in the table, the annual probability of death for all causes is just below one for all causes. To calculate the overall likelihood of dying each year, one must multiply the individual probabilities with each other[198]. This results in a probability of 0.9923. A man who turns 80 has faced this annual risk 80 times. Calculating the probability that a man can celebrate his 80th birthday, one must multiply 0.9923 with itself 80 times; $0.9923*0.9923*0.99238*...*0.9923 = 0.9923^{80} = 0.5388$.

Cause of death	Deaths per 100,000	Annual probability of death
Heart disease	173.8	0.9983
Cancer	146.6	0.9985
COVID-19	104.1	0.999
Unintentional injuries	64.7	0.9994
Stroke	41.1	0.9996
Chronic lower respiratory disease	34.7	0.9997
Alzheimer	31	0.9997
Diabetes	25.4	0.9997
Chronic liver disease and cirrhosis	14.5	0.9999
Kidney disease	13.6	0.9999
Others*	140	0.9986
Overall annual probability of death:		0.9923
Probability of reaching your 80th birthday as a male**:		0.5388

[197] Data from 2021 sourced from: https://www.cdc.gov/

[198] For simplicity, dependencies between diseases have been ignored.

Table 9.1. The ten most common fatal diseases in the US.
* This number was chosen to ensure that the probability of a male reaching his 80th year corresponds to 54%. ** $0.9923^{80} = 0.5388$

Figure 9.6 shows how the percentage of males that are still alive drops with time. The figure assumes a constant rate of death.

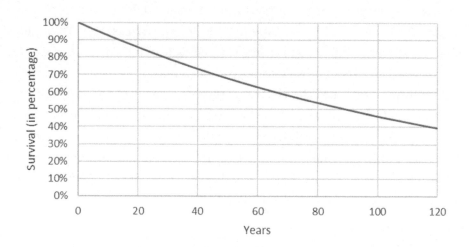

Figure 9.6. Survival assuming a constant rate of death.

The point of this exercise is to demonstrate that a probability that is only slightly smaller than 100% will result in a probability that is significantly smaller than 100% if these high probabilities are multiplied many times over.

The assumption of a constant death rate is obviously not true. It is ridiculous to assume that 40% of males have a lifespan exceeding 120 years. True life is a lot more interesting. This will be discussed in the following section.

Human survival statistics

[Difficulty: Blue]

The question 'how many much time have I left?' is impossible to answer. Life is per definition finite – we are all going to die one day. However, the day on which we die is inherently uncertain.

Jeanne Louise Calment was the oldest person who ever lived, until she died at the age of 122 years. It has been reported that she was in good health, though almost blind and deaf[199]. The oldest person alive today is Lucile Randon. Lucile is blind and has been wheelchair-bound since the early 2010s. When Lucile became the world's oldest living person, she stated that this was a "sad honour" as she would "be better off in heaven"[200].

Survival curves describe the development of the mortality rate over time. In other words, it describes the trend in the probability of surviving another year as we age. We can study survival rates using Kaplan–Meier curves. A Kaplan–Meier (K-M) curve starts at 100% at time 0 and decreases to 0% as time progresses. This step function is a key characteristic of a K-M curve. Each step approximates the true survival rate at a particular time.

Survival rates[201], i.e., the chance of surviving another year, increase until people reach their early twenties. At that point, a slow exponential decline set in, and this decline persists until people reach their early 80s. Differences between males and females become increasingly pronounced during this long period of exponential decline (Figure 9.7)[202]. The differences between the sexes increase to a maximum of almost 14% when humans reach their 84th year.

---

[199] https://en.wikipedia.org/wiki/Jeanne_Calment

[200] https://en.wikipedia.org/wiki/Lucile_Randon

[201] The survival rate should not be confused with the mortality rate. Survival and mortality are each other's opposite: Survival Rate = (1 − Mortality Rate). Source: https://www. cdc.gov/nchs/data/nvsr/nvsr68/nvsr68_07-508.pdf

[202] If you ask any 80-year-old, they will assure you that their life went by way too fast.

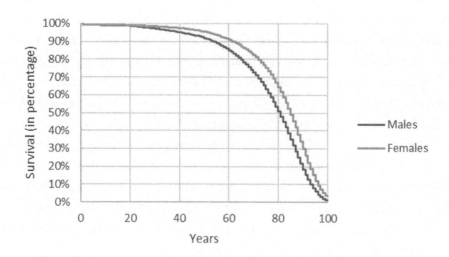

Figure 9.7. Male and female general population survival curves.

Beyond the age of 80, both males' and females' survival rates start to decline rapidly. It is difficult to obtain a complete picture of the survival curve. As we move down the survival curve, there is fewer and less data to support the shape of the survival curve. In addition to having fewer data points available, there is a secondary trend that complicates matters: the current generation is outliving previous generations. The cause of death is changing. We are living longer today than we did 100 years ago because of advances in medical science and improved sanitation, nutrition, and hygiene. Just over a century ago, the average life expectancy at birth for a man was 48.4 years, whereas women could expect to live to 54.0 years. Fast forward from 1915 to 2015, and a man's life span extended by 31 years and a woman's by almost 29 years (79.3 and 82.9, respectively). This complication adds another layer of uncertainty when analysing survival data.

Because survival data apply to a large population size, its estimates are very accurate. For example, the statement '50% of males live to the age of 80 years' can be made with a high degree of confidence because the data collected indicate that about half of the males died before reaching this age. This statement is

245

referred to as a *prognosis*[203]. This prognosis refers to an average male, i.e., the only information available to us is the fact that we are dealing with a male. This statistical information does not apply to an individual male because characteristics specific to the individual can substantially change the expected life span. Additional information is needed to determine whether a male's life span is more likely to exceed 80 years. For example, if we had some data on this individual that gave us confidence that we were dealing with a healthy man.

A different way of interpreting survival curves can be achieved by replotting the data and investigating the probability of dying within a given year, i.e., the survival data is turned into a discrete probability distribution (Figure 9.8). The fact that we are investigating proper probabilities implies that the area under the curve should always equal 1[204]. The total of 1 is reflective of the only certainty we have in life – sooner or later we will all die.

The shape of the probability distribution changes as a person ages. The survival curve of a 14-year-old male is very different from that of an 80-year-old male. The probability that an 80-year-old male dies within a year is approximately 5%, whereas the probability that a 14-year-old male dies within the same period is 0.023%. The ratio between these two probabilities is approximately 200.

The second aspect that really stands out is the difference in the expected remaining life years. A randomly chosen 80-year-old male has about a 1.5% chance of surviving 20 more years. A 14-year-old male has at least a 97% chance of surviving 20 more years.

---

[203] A prognosis is not to be confused with a diagnosis. A diagnosis refers to the process of identifying a disease from its symptoms. A prognosis is an opinion on the most likely development of a disease. I am not sure in this particular case whether ageing qualifies as a disease – maybe life is a disease…

[204] 1 is this context equals 100%.

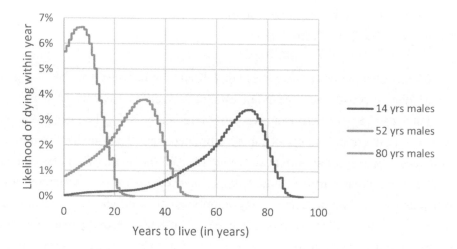

Figure 9.8. Three probability distributions of generations of males. My Dad, who turned 80 this year; our son, who is 14 years old; and me, who is 52 years old.

The three selected ages shown in Figure 9.8 were not randomly chosen. Our son is 14 years old, my Dad is 80 years old and I am 52 years old. Three generations of males in the same family. All three have a very different outlook on life. Our son is a completely healthy young lad and there is a high probability that he still has much time left to enjoy his life. My Dad has taken many pain medications over a large portion of his life, and I know that he did not expect to reach his 9th decade of being alive. Given my illness, from the three of us, it is very likely that I will be the first to die.

Survival analysis in clinical trials

[Difficulty: Black]

There are three main ways of analysing the outcomes of a clinical trial[205]:

- Reporting the median survival for each treatment arm;

---

[205] In the literature, clinical trials are referred as Randomised Clinical Trials or RCTs.

- Time point analyses (e.g., proportion of patients alive at 1 and 5 years for each treatment arm[206]) and;
- The hazard ratio (HR).

Claims of superiority[207] are based on HR and median survival[208].

Median survival and time point estimates, such as 1- or 5-year survival, estimates can be generated from Kaplan–Meier analysis[209]. The magnitude and direction of the treatment effect can be estimated from these medians and point estimates[210]. The most important and objective endpoint in many cancers clinical trials is the median survival time. Comparing medians for each treatment arm provides an absolute measure of any improvement in efficacy (e.g., 2 months difference in the median survival) relative to a particular absolute median for the control group. Other absolute measures of improved efficacy between the treatment arms include the proportion of patients surviving at defined time points (e.g., such as 1-year Overall Survival probability). Two types of survival time are generally recorded; Overall Survival which is the time to death and Progression Free Survival which is the time to disease recurrence or progression of tumour growth.

The hazard ratio (HR) summarises all the information in the entire K-M survival curve into a single number. HR provides an estimate of the relative efficacy between the treatment arms. A simplistic interpretation is that a HR = 1 means an equal efficacy of the experimental and standard of care (Figure 9.9). Usually, the HR is presented so that if the experimental treatment is (i) better than the standard of care then the HR <1 or (ii) worse than the standard of care then the HR >1.

---

[206] This is statistically justified because the two groups of patients are being randomised before treatment starts. This is fundamentally different from the scenario described in the section *Five-year survival and mortality: Giuliani's prostate cancer.*

[207] Better performing, equally good or non-inferior

[208] Barraclough et al., 2011.

[209] Kaplan and Meier, 1958.

[210] Barraclough et al., 2011.

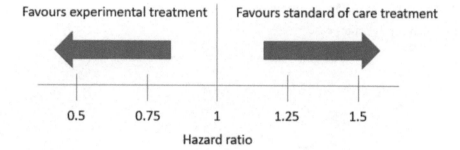

Figure 9.9. Visualisation of the hazard ratio (HR). HR equals 1 if the experimental drug and standard of care have the same efficacy. If the experimental treatment is better than the standard of care, then the HR <1. If the experimental treatment is worse than the standard of care, then HR >1.

For example, in the case of Overall Survival, the implication of a HR that is equal to 0.75 is a 25% lower risk of death on the experimental treatment than the control. The experimental treatment is usually a novel drug, and the control group is another treatment or a placebo.

The HR is usually calculated from a Cox proportional hazard model, which is one of the standard methods for analysing survival end points in oncology Randomised Clinical Trials. The Cox proportional hazard regression analysis is a very useful technique because it allows one to determine HRs while adjusting for other factors that might influence the risk for age, sex, educational level, occupational class, smoking, and physical activity. Although you do not really need to understand the details behind Cox regression, one should be aware that one of the assumptions of the regression modelling is that the hazard ratio is kept constant over time[211].

Mode, median, and mean

[Difficulty: Blue]

If you asked me to give you a single number, what number would you ask for? Here are some options available to you (Figure 9.10):

---

[211] Spotswood et al., 2004.

Mode (or most likely) case;

The median (or P50 or fiftieth percentage) case and;

Mean (or average) case.

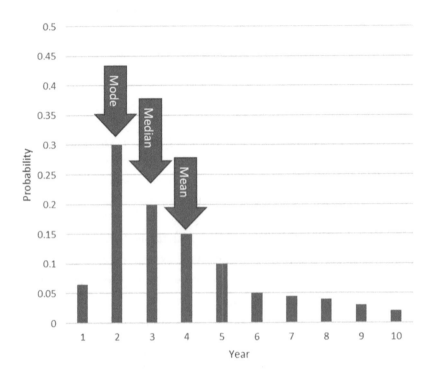

Figure 9.10. A distribution that has a different value for the mean, median, and mode.

All these options have different statistical meanings. If you increase the asymmetry of the distribution, the difference between the mode, median, and mean will increase. I am not sure that if you are asking for survival times, the mean is the most insightful number. By not using the mean value, I diverge from the consensus view of my fellow decision analysts. The optimal strategy when making many decisions can be achieved by consistently choosing the mean value[212]. However, when dealing with skewed distributions, i.e., asymmetric distributions, the mean will be controlled by a few very extreme values. I am also not a fan of this mode, aka as the most likely case. The mode of the distribution

---

[212] An infinite number of decisions is required for the solution to converge to the optimal strategy.

does not provide any insight apart from the fact that it is the most likely single value.

I would settle on the median. The median, also known as the 50th percentage or the P50, splits the distribution in half. Half of the numbers are smaller than the median and the other half are larger than the median.

In a discussion about survival time with your doctor, ensure you ask for the median!

Rather than focussing on a single number, one could also ask for the complete set of numbers and calculate summary values that provide insight into the overall distribution of possible outcomes.

Confidence intervals

[Difficulty: Black]

David Spiegelhalter starts chapter nine of his book *The Art of Statistics* with a warning: *'This is perhaps the most challenging [part] of this book but persevering with this important topic will give a valuable insight into statistical inference.'* I highly recommend reading his book. Particularly if you get confused by what follows below[213].

Confidence intervals are an important part of the communication of statistical information. Most statistical measures described in this book are uncertain. Means, odds ratios, hazard ratios, and relative risk are all inherently uncertain. The variability in these statistics can be described by a probability distribution. A probability distribution is nothing more than a quantification of the uncertainty of the statistic.

Moving from a discrete distribution to a standard normal distribution

Two types of probability distributions exist: discrete and continuous. A discrete probability distribution consists of a set of values, generally referred to as buckets, that each have been assigned a probability value. Per definition, the total sum across all buckets adds to 1. Figure 9.11 shows an example of the probability distribution, in this case a discrete version of a normal distribution.

---

[213] I believe it is very insightful reading several descriptions of the same topic as authors use different words to explain an identical concept.

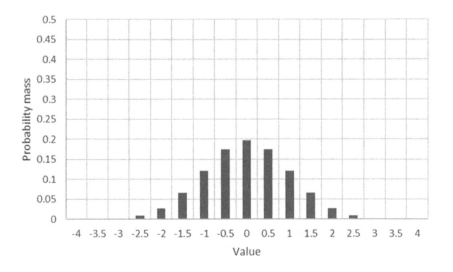

Figure 9.11. Discrete normal probability distribution.

In Figure 9.11, the width of the individual bucket is 0.5. We can reduce the width of the bucket from 0.5 to 0.4 and then to 0.1. If we proceed this way, we ultimately end up with a bucket width that is infinitesimal small, i.e., the width is zero. Once that has been achieved, a continuous distribution has been created. The vertical bars have been replaced with a bell-shaped curve that defines the normal distribution[214].

Continuous probability distributions are different from discrete probability distributions in the sense that an infinite number of points, or "buckets", have been defined over a continuous interval. Therefore, the probability for a single value is always – per definition – zero.

A probability density function defines the shape of the probability distributions. There are many types of probability density functions. In many cases the process underlying the randomness defines what probability function is most appropriate to use. For example, when adding numbers, a normal distribution is appropriate to use and when one multiplies numbers a lognormal distribution is appropriate.

---

[214] In discrete probability distributions, we discuss probability mass, and in continuous distributions, we discuss probability density.

A key property shared among all probability density functions is that the area underneath the curve has a value of 1. As the values plotted along the horizontal axis show the full range of possible values, the sum of the probabilities of all these possible values must be 1.

Confidence intervals, the topic discussed below, require normalised normal distributions. Normalising a normal distribution is easy; simply set the mean equal to 0 and set the standard deviation to 1: $N(\mu = 0, \sigma = 1)$.

Confidence intervals

In a continuous distribution, a bucket must be defined by choosing a lower and upper limit of the value that is plotted along the horizontal axis. These limits, represented by two vertical lines from the probability density function down to the horizontal axis, define the area underneath the curve (Figure 9.12). The size of this area underneath the curve is equal to the probability that a random value is obtained between these two limits.

How do we set these upper and lower limits? The normal distribution is defined by two metrics: the mean and the standard deviation. The mean is the value that you would expect to find. When sampling a normal distribution many times, the best bet is to assume that the sampled value equals the mean. The standard deviation is a measure of variability. Loosely speaking, the standard deviation refers to the width of a normal distribution. The smaller the standard deviation, the narrower the normal distribution becomes as the degree of variability is reduced. The larger the standard deviation, the wider the distribution becomes as the degree of variability increases.

It is common practise for statisticians to report a range limited by a multiple of the standard deviation that is centred around the mean. For example, 3.92 standard deviations centred around the mean has a probability, or an area underneath the curve, of 95% (Table 9.2, Figure 9.12).

These ranges of a multiple of standard deviation centred around the mean are commonly referred to as confidence intervals, error ranges, or confidence ranges. Commonly used intervals include 99%, 95%, 90%, and 80%. Table 9.2 lists the width of the interval, the lower limit, the upper limit, and the number of standard deviations between the mean and the lower or upper limits of the interval[215].

---

[215] This analysis assumes a mean of zero and a standard deviation of one.

Confidence interval	Number of standard deviations	Lower limit	Upper limit
0.8	1.282	0.1	0.9
0.9	1.645	0.05	0.95
0.95	1.96	0.025	0.975
0.99	2.576	0.005	0.995

Table 9.2. Four commonly used confidence intervals.

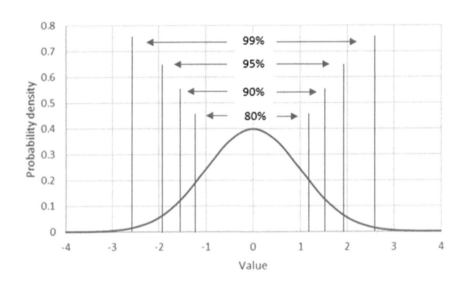

Figure 9.12. A normal distribution with four confidence intervals.

Central Limit Theorem

The Central Limit Theorem dictates that regardless of the shape of the original distribution, the distribution converges to a normal distribution with an increased sample size[216]. In other words, once you take a large number of samples from the original distribution those sampled values will resemble a normal distribution.

A fundamental property of the normal distribution is its symmetry. The mean, median, and mode all have the same values, and you can flip the distribution vertically along its mean without any effect. The resulting distribution will have all the same characteristics as before the flipping operation.

---

[216] An exception would be if a distribution has no mean to converge to.

Given these properties, it is common practice to define the symmetrical confidence interval around the mean.

The Central Limit Theorem allows for an approximation when adding random variable by using a normal random variable. This is extremely useful because it is normally much easier to deal with normal distributions than other probability distributions.

The next section demonstrates the Central Limit Theorem, as well as the Law of Large Numbers, by means of a die rolling example.

The Law of Large Numbers

As the sample size increases, the shape of the distribution also changes. It gradually becomes narrower, i.e., the variability in the statistic decreases. This phenomenon is referred to as the Law of Large Numbers.

The principle of the Law of Large Numbers can be illustrated by rolling a die. For this type of experiment, the binomial process is appropriate. "Success" is defined by having thrown a *six*. The chance of success for a single experiment, i.e., one throw of the die of a six-sided unweighted die, is $^1/_6$ (Upper left panel of Figure 9.13). In the following experiment, a die is rolled ten times. The probability that none of the throws yields a *six* is reduced from 83%[217] to 16%[218], whereas the probability of throwing a single *six* is increased from 17% to 32% (Upper two panels of Figure 9.13). The probability of throwing more than 6 *sixes* is far less than 0.3%, i.e., rapidly approaching zero.

The trend of reducing the probability of throwing null successes, i.e., no *sixes*, and reducing the probability of throwing all successes, i.e., all *sixes*, continuous if we repeat the experiment 100 and 1000 times. Another related observation we can make, when comparing all four scenarios, is that the distribution progressively becomes more like a normal distribution. By repeating binomial sampling many times, we find a result that has the properties of a normal distribution. The fact that a binomial distribution becomes a normal distribution has profound implications. Because this transition is true for the vast majority of probability distributions, this rule can be generally applied. This rule is known as the Law of Large Numbers.

---

[217] In the single throw experiment.

[218] In the experiment with 10 rolls of the die.

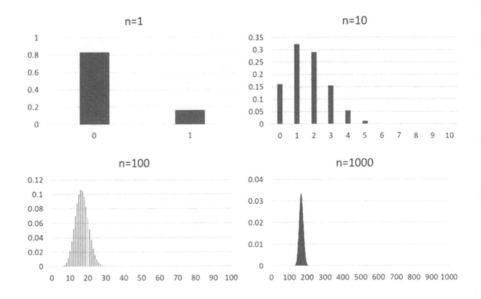

Figure 9.13. Rolling a die once, ten times, hundred times, and a thousand times.

There are two implications of the Law of Large Numbers; 1) The mean of the underlying distribution is close to the average of many independent samples. 2) The density histogram of many independent samples converges to the density of the underlying distribution.

The importance of being precise

Interpretation of the precise meaning of a confidence interval is actually very difficult to comprehend. This is an understatement – many generations of students of statistics have been baffled, and I have no reason to believe that will change any time soon. Are you ready?

Here it is: A 95% confidence interval in a frequentist sense is defined as if one takes a random sample that the statistic, e.g., the sample mean, has a 95% chance of falling into this range[219].

If you are confused, you are in good company, as most of us were confused after reading this statement for the first time!

---

[219] I was offered the following definition by a colleague, who actually has a PhD in statistics: 'I prefer to think of repeating the random sample many times and calculating a confidence interval each time. 95% of these intervals will contain the true value'.

The relevance of this precise definition is that is tempting to think that there is a 95% probability that a value falls into the defined range, but this is not necessarily true. For example, when considering a medical test. Although it is true that 95% of people taking the test get the correct result, the converse is not necessarily true, i.e., that 95% of the positive tests are true.

Systematic errors

A systematic error or bias will skew the reported results. These errors can result from the way the data were collected. For example, in the prediction of election results, people's data are collected using landlines (Spiegelhalter, 2019). The use of landlines might introduce a bias. As certain people (e.g., young voters) do not use landlines any longer. The data collected is not a representative sample of all voters; it is skewed towards people who have access to a landline.

The survival data used in the assessment of the length of my remaining life also has multiple biases. Two predicting factors of survival in glioblastoma patients are age and MGMT[220] status. Older patients have a poorer life outlook than younger patients; therefore, ideally, one would like to correct for age[221]. This leaves me with the question of whether I am a true representative sample of the cohort of patients suffering from glioblastoma.

Type 1 and Type 2 errors and the power of a clinical study

The Federal Drug Administration (FDA) in the USA and the European Medicines Agency (EMA) in Europe are tasked with the approval of novel drugs. A key requirement of new drugs is that they must have an effect. A drug should have a certain level of efficacy. Statistics are used to develop evidence for the efficacy of a novel drug. This is done by developing a hypothesis. A hypothesis is a statement of the outcome of a study. A null hypothesis and an alternative hypothesis are typically developed as follows:

---

[220] MGMT status is related to the expression of an enzyme involved in DNA repair. Methylation is a chemical reaction involving a methyl group that is added to DNA. In doing so, the DNA sequence cannot produce any proteins.

[221] One could attempt to apply a correction using Cox regression.

1. The null hypothesis states that there is no difference between the treatments in terms of benefits.
2. The alternative hypothesis states that there is a difference between the treatments in terms of benefits.

Once these two hypotheses are defined and the study has been completed, a statistical test is performed to determine whether the observed differences are statistically significant. Clearly, there is no such thing as certainty in statistics. Hence, the concept of confidence intervals is being applied. The data collected in the study is used to express how confident we are in the null hypotheses and the alternative hypothesis. A 95% confidence interval is a common choice (see previous section). As there is no certainty that there is room for error, there is a probability that a mistake is made. Two types of errors can occur: Type 1 and Type 2 errors. There are four possible outcomes, two of which are false (Figure 9.14).

Actual truth

		Treatment benefit	No treatment benefit
Clinical trial result	Treatment benefit	Correct result	Type 1 error (False positive)
	No treatment benefit	Type 2 error (False negative)	Correct result

Figure 9.14 The four feasible outcomes.

A type 1 error occurs when we incorrectly reject the null hypothesis (the null hypothesis is true, but the clinical trial indicates that there is a treatment benefit). For example, in one of the TMZ studies, Malmström et al. (2012) states: 'hazard ratio [HR] 0·70; 95% CI 0·52-0·93, p=0·01.' In plain English this means that a hazard ratio of 0.70 has been observed, the 95% confidence interval extends from 0.52 to 0.92, and finally that the probability that a Type 1 error has been made is 1%.

A type 2 error occurs when we incorrectly accept the null hypothesis (the alternative hypothesis is true, but the clinical trial indicates that there is a no treatment benefit)[222]. The power of a clinical trial is a measure that quantifies the avoidance of a type 2 error. The power of a clinical trial is the probability that the study will detect a predetermined difference in measurement between the two groups, given the chosen confidence interval and sample size, i.e., the number of patients.

Relative risk

[Difficulty: Blue]

To aid the understanding of percentages Figure 9.15 shows a visual representation of percentages. Each panel shows 100 squares in two shades of blue. The darker blue marks a different proportion in each of the panels, as indicated by percentage. You can see that 50% is completely different from 10% and 10% is completely different from 1%.

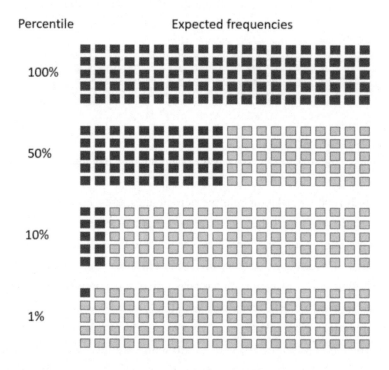

Figure 9.15. Visual representation of percentages.

---

[222] Jones et al., 2003.

There is a different and possibly more effective way of showing these percentages by randomising the squares before showing them (Figure 9.16).

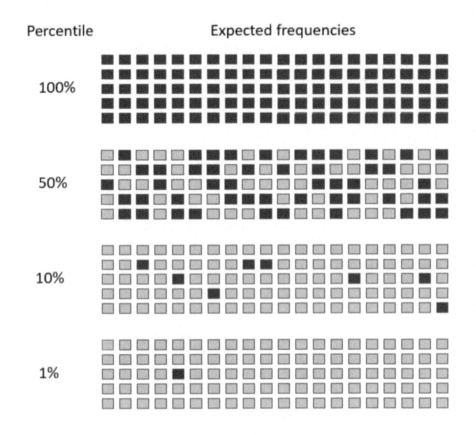

Figure 9.16. The same percentages but now randomised.

Although relative risks, or relative percentages, are one of the most natural and least confusing of all the measures of treatment effect in clinical trials[223], both patients and doctors are confused by relative risks. The lower two panels illustrate that 10% and 1% are very different, although both assessments can be characterised as extreme events. The relative difference between 10% and 1% is as large as the relative difference between 100% and 10%. If a future event has 100% probability of happening, there is no uncertainty. It is a fact. When you multiply 10% by a factor of 10, you end up with certainty, whereas if you were to divide 10% by the same number, you end up with 1% – a probability that is

---

[223] Case et al., 2002.

significantly more extreme but is still of the same category, i.e., an extreme value. Both 10% and 1% are considered to be extreme values.

Relative risks work if the calculated value is less than 100%. In situations where the upper value exceeds 100%, the logic breaks down. Doubling 49% yields 98%. At 98%, there is still a level of uncertainty, as this value is lower than 100%. Doubling 51% yields 102%. This answer is a non-sensible percentage, as it exceeds 100%. Doubling 50% yields 100%. There is no uncertainty at 100%; therefore, even this value has some nonsensible attributes.

Other examples are known to science where further extrapolation yields nonsensible results: south of the South Pole and black holes. It is impossible to go further south once you reach the South Pole[224]. No matter what direction you choose, you will end up going north. Inside a black hole, time has come to a standstill. Hence, the concept of time has no meaning inside a black hole.

The issue described above is not symmetrical. One can always divide the percentage. The percentage obtained will be smaller but will always be a positive number. Trouble sets in when you start multiplying a percentage with a value greater than 1.

An example of relative risk

[Difficulty: Red]

Assume that a company is interested in investigating the effect of a new oncology drug that is expected to have a beneficial effect on Overall Survival[225]. A clinical trial was designed where the effect of the drug was compared in two groups of 100 patients. At the end of the trial, we might have the following situation. In the group that received the drug, 92 people survived the trial, compared with 90 survivors in the group that received treatment following current treatment guidelines (Table 9.3). The latter treatment is generally referred to as the Standard of Care (SoC).

---

[224] Well, unless you launch a rocket and travel in space southwards!

[225] No pharmaceutical company will use this trial design. The sole purpose of this example is to illustrate the calculation of statistics with some simple numbers.

Treatment	Dead patients	Living patients
1	8	92
2	10	90

Table 9.3. Response by treatment.

The risk of dying during treatment 1 equals to $p_1 = \dfrac{Number\ of\ dead\ patients}{Total\ number\ of\ patients} =$ $\dfrac{8}{100} = 0.08 = 8\%$; the equivalent calculation for treatment 2 yields a percentage of 10%.

The relative risk is defined as:

$$Relative\ risk =$$
$$\dfrac{Number\ of\ dead\ patients\ treatment\ 1\Big/Total\ number\ of\ patients\ receiving\ treatment\ 1}{Number\ of\ dead\ patients\ treatment\ 2\Big/Total\ number\ of\ patients\ receiving\ treatment\ 2}$$

$$= \dfrac{8/100}{10/100} = 0.8 = 80\%$$

There is a widespread misconception that this 80% reduction implies that 80 out of 100 patients will be saved by the treatment, i.e., people interpret a relative risk as an absolute percentage (Figure 9.17). The absolute percentage is simply the difference between 10% and 8%. In absolute percentages, the improvement is 2%. This difference is much less impressive than the 80% relative percentile difference reported previously.

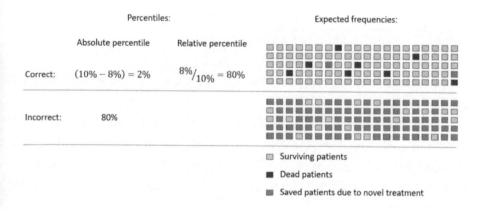

Figure 9.17. Two correct interpretations in the top panel and an incorrect interpretation in the middle panel.

Using the absolute difference, it is easy to calculate the Number Needed to Treat. This number refers to the number of patients who require treatment to save one life. In this scenario, two of 100 patients can be saved by this treatment. Therefore, if the treatment is provided to 50 patients, one life will be saved. The Number Needed to Treat is 50. Although the Number Needed to Treat was introduced as an easy-to-understand and therefore useful metric, several subsequent studies have pointed out that there are some fundamental issues with this method[226].

Finally, because the relative risk is a relative measure, an increase in response from 8% to 10% gives the same relative risk as an increase from 80% to 100%. Despite the fact that these two results are fundamentally different. A trial in which 8% of the participants die is very different from a trial in which 80% of the participating patients die.

Odds and Odds Ratio

[Difficulty: Black]

Another two metrics that cause confusion are the Odds and the Odds Ratio.

Odds

The Odds are defined by:

---

[226] Altman, 1998; Grieve, 2003 and Wald, 2020.

$$Odds = \frac{deceased\ patients}{total\ number\ of\ patients - deceased\ patients} = \frac{x}{(X - x)}$$

where x represents the number of deceased patients and X represents the total number of patients.

Odds is not a probability. As the denominator is not equal to "the total number of patients" but "the total number of patients minus the deceased patients", the Odds are – per definition – a higher number. The Odds number is used to assess the likelihood that a patient with a certain condition will develop a certain illness.

We can rewrite the Odds equation as:

$$Odds = \frac{p}{(1 - p)}$$

where p is the percentage of deceased patients.

For example, if the probability of an event is 0.2, the Odds of that event is $0.2/0.8 = 0.25$, or 1 to 4. Figure 9.18 shows how the difference between the percentage and Odds vary. For low percentage values, the difference is small, but for higher percentages, the difference becomes large – in fact, infinite when the percentage is set at 100%.

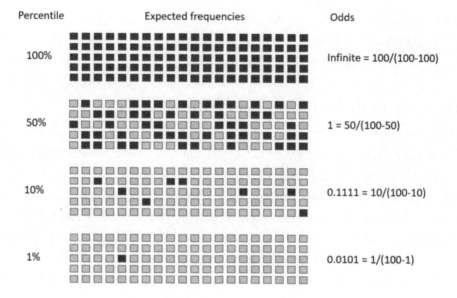

Percentile	Expected frequencies	Odds
100%		Infinite = 100/(100-100)
50%		1 = 50/(100-50)
10%		0.1111 = 10/(100-10)
1%		0.0101 = 1/(100-1)

Figure 9.18. Difference between Odds and percentage.

Odds Ratio

The next concept to be introduced is the Odds Ratio. The Odds Ratio is the ratio between the Odds of treatment 1, denote by $Odds_1$:

$$Odds_1 = {p_1}/{(1 - p_1)}$$

An equivalent calculation can be used to determine the $Odds_2$:

$$Odds_2 = {p_2}/{(1 - p_2)}$$

The formula to determine the Odds ratio is as follows:

$$Odds\ Ratio = \frac{{p_1}/{(1 - p_1)}}{{p_2}/{(1 - p_2)}} = \frac{p_1(1 - p_2)}{p_2(1 - p_1)}$$

The measure of association is the same as the Odds Ratio or its reciprocal[227]. This symmetry led some statisticians to suggest that Odds Ratio should be the gold standard[228]. Others disagree, judging the Odds Ratio to be an incomprehensible number[229].

On the importance of clear definitions

[Difficulty: Red]

Misinterpretations can lead to an overestimation of the clinical effect. For example, interpreting the probability as an Odds ratio would lead to such overestimation of clinical benefits. It is important, given the ubiquity of statistical models for analysing response and survival in cancer clinical trials, that measures such as Odd Ratios and Hazard Ratios be clearly understood, lest we misstate the benefit of clinical treatments. This is particularly relevant for physicians, who must communicate the statistical findings of cancer clinical trials using words that their patients can understand[230].

We should be mindful that there is a bias towards publishing positive trial results[231]. It is therefore not surprising that several studies have demonstrated how the results can be manipulated to exaggerate the effect of a new treatment[232], and there are even studies that demonstrate how a single data set can lead to opposite conclusions[233].

Definition of risk

In the summer of 2007, I gave a presentation in Aberdeen just after I started working for Palantir Economic Solutions. We invited all clients and some potential clients for an afternoon session where we presented our latest product

---

[227] The product of the Odds Ratio and the inverse of the Odds Ratio is 1.

[228] Case et al., 2002.

[229] Lee, 1994.

[230] Case et al., 2002.

[231] Pocock, 1983.

[232] e.g. Pocock and Stone, 2016.

[233] e.g. Baar and Tannock, 1989.

offering: a real option model[234]. I remember walking onto the stage and showing the first slide. It took 45 minutes before I moved on to my second slide. I was dragged into a discussion about what I meant by the word *"risk"*. I will never forget how passionate people are about their favourite definition of the word *risk*. I was in a room filled with economists and business development people, and between us, at least 10 different definitions of risk were named: technical risk, market risk, private risk, credit risk, liquidity risk, operational risk, value-at-risk, risk attitude, audit risk, safety risk, etc. All these definitions of risk are related to the possibility of something bad happening. Risks involve negative things happening to something that is valued by people. Risk refers to the negative impact on people's health, well-being, wealth, or property. Risk also refers to negative environmental developments. In all these examples, risk focuses on negative, undesirable consequences. Some people define risk as being an uncertainty. Risk, in their opinion, can be both positive and negative.

I thought our clients were attending for the free lunch; clearly not!

What I learned that day is that it is really important to have a clear definition of the words you are using and do not assume that your definition is the same as the person you are having a conversation with.

Does screening for cancer save lives?

[Difficulty: Red]

'I had prostate cancer five, six years ago', Mr Giuliani, a Republican presidential candidate, said in a speech that has been turned into a radio commercial. 'My chance of surviving prostate cancer – and, thank God, I was cured of it – in the United States? Eighty-two per cent. What is my chance of surviving prostate cancer in England? Only 44 % under socialised medicine.'

Eighty-two per cent versus forty-four per the cent: can "socialise medicine" make such a large difference?

The real reason for the difference is the fact that cancer screening is much more common in the United States than in the United Kingdom. In the United States, prostate cancer tends to be found earlier simply because if you find it earlier. Hence, you will always have longer survival after the disease is

---

[234] The concept of real options is no longer *in vogue,* but it used to be a hot topic in the late 1990s or early 2000s. In its most basic formulation, the assumption is made that oil prices would follow a Brownian motion.

diagnosed early. All physicians should know that these figures tell us nothing about whether screening actually saves lives. Differences in 5-year survival rates do not correlate with differences in mortality rates[235].

Cancer can be diagnosed by either symptoms or screening. Screening detects cancer before it causes any symptoms. Because of this property, screening can bias 5-year survival rates in 2 ways: 1) by prolonging the period in which patients are known to have cancer and 2) by including people with nonprogressive cancer in the statistic. The first, called *lead-time bias*, accounts for the fact that screening may only reduce the time to diagnosis without increasing the time to death. This prolonged period of diagnosis makes patients attending screening more likely to be included in the 5-year survival statistic. However, this may have no bearing on real prolonged or saved lives[236]. The second phenomenon, called *length-time bias* or *overdiagnosis bias*, concerns the detection of lesions that meet the pathological definition of cancer but never become clinically significant because of their slow growth[237].

One study[238] gave 65 physicians the actual changes in 5-year survival rates from the Surveillance, Epidemiology and End Result (SEER) programme for prostate cancer, which showed differences similar to those reported by Giuliani. Considering the 5-year survival rates, 78% of doctors judged the screening as effective. Only 2 of the 65 physicians understood the lead time bias and not a single physician understood the overdiagnosis bias.

If these numbers are confusing the following example might be easier to comprehend. Imagine two tests. The first test reduces the risk of dying from 1% to 0%. The second test reduces the risk of death from 5% to 2%. Which test would you take: the first or the second? If you think like most people, you will opt for the first test. This preference is also known as the *Zero-risk fallacy*. The first test provides certainty, and there is zero risk. However, the second test is preferable as it offers a 3% reduction as opposed to just 1% offered by the first test.

The bottom line is that it is very hard to establish whether screening actually saves lives. Even if we could accurately assess the benefits of screening, we would still be faced with biases that affect our judgement.

---

[235] Welch et al., 2000; Li et al., 2017.

[236] Gordis, 2008.

[237] Wegwarth et al, 2011.

[238] Wegwarth et al., 2011.

Concluding remarks: Innumeracy

Statistics, such as the mean and the standard deviation, summarise and characterise the real world. Statistics create insight and aid communication of the complexity present in our surroundings. The confusion that arises when we do not fully understand the meaning of the reported statistics makes us vulnerable to misguidance and manipulation.

The systematic explanation of the most commonly used statistical measures should have improved your understanding of your situation.

The purpose of the following chapter, *Human judgement*, is to teach the reader the skills to acquire objective judgements and mitigate the effect of biases.

Appendix: Standard Deviation and Standard Error

Standard deviation

[Difficulty: Black]

$$Standard\ deviation = \sigma = \sqrt{\frac{\Sigma(x_i - \mu)^2}{n - 1}}$$

Where x represents the value of sample i,
μ represents the sample mean and
n equals to the number of samples.
Note that $n - 1$ is the correction for the degrees of freedom.

Standard error

[Difficulty: Black]
Variability in statistics is based on samples

$$Standard\ Error = SE = \frac{\sigma}{\sqrt{(n - 1)}}$$

Where σ represents the sample standard deviation and
n equals to the number of samples

Human Judgement

'Complexity is the hallmark of life [and the brain] involves about 10^{29} particles and is mind-blowingly complex.'

Tegmark in *Our Mathematical Universe*

'I regard it a triumph that we, who are ourselves mere stardust, have come to such detailed understanding of the universe in which we live.'

Stephen Hawking in *Brief Answers to Big Questions*

Abstract Human Judgement

The human brain appears to have two modes of creating judgements. Although this dualism was already recognised in the 17th century by Descartes, it was not until the 21st century that Kahneman labelled the default thinking mode as System 1 and the more methodical thinking mode as System 2.

System 1 requires a small amount of cognitive resources, cannot be stopped voluntarily, and occurs unconsciously. System 1 creates believable stories. System 1 distort reality by simplifying the world around us. Psychologists refer to these distortions of reality as *biases*. Many biases have been identified, and the most important biases are described in this chapter. System 2 requires a considerable amount of cognitive resources, can be stopped voluntarily, and occurs consciously. System 2 is our rationale for creating judgements. System 2 is used to think through a problem by conscious analysis.

System 1 is exposed to rule-of-thumb (heuristic) biases that are often predictable. Because of their predictability, it is possible to mitigate biases through careful questioning. The process of collecting judgements is referred to as expert elicitation.

Two systems of thinking

[Difficulty: Blue]

Descartes' mind-body dualism, published in the seventeenth century, first raised the notion that there are two fundamentally different ways to construct a judgement. The foundation for *System 1* and *System 2* thinking was developed by William James, an American psychologist, in *Principles of Psychology*.

James argued that associative knowledge is derived from past experiences as opposed to true reasoning being used in new, unfamiliar scenarios.

In *Thinking, Fast, and Slow,* Kahneman defines the default thinking mode as System 1 and the more methodical thinking mode as System 2. System 1 works instantly and creates believable stories. I explained my collapse in the garden as a logical chain of events. I ignored the clues that there was something seriously wrong with me.

In the same book, Daniel Kahneman summarises several decades of psychological research and discusses how people create judgements. Richard Thaler's book *Nudge* describes how people's behaviour can be changed predictably. Both authors have been awarded the Nobel Prize in Economic Sciences. These two books, *Thinking, Fast and Slow* and *Nudge,* changed public perception of the relevance of psychology to practical decision-making.

Pattern recognition features extensively in *Blink* by Malcolm Gladwell. He gives an example of a firefighter entering a room but stepping back after a fraction of a second because something did not feel right. His hunch was confirmed a few moments later as the floor on which he had been standing collapsed. It turned out that the fire originated in the basement, not on the ground floor.

Humans should think fast in situations where time is of the essence. You don't want to spend hours analysing the sound you heard behind you. Once you recognise that the sound originates from a car engine, you immediately jump out of the way.

Chess Grandmaster Magnus Carlsen once told a journalist that he would find the best move by glancing at a chess board for only a few seconds. This illustrates System 1 and the role of pattern recognition at the Grandmaster level. After System 1 informs Magnus Carlsen of the optimal move, he will spend the next 10 to 20 minutes checking whether that particular move is indeed the best move. That is System 2 thinking. Sometimes it is obvious when you should switch to System 2. For example, to determine the answer to a complex question:

True or false: $23*14>27*12$

You know that you will have to work it out with a pen and paper.

In some cases, it is obvious that System 1 is sufficient:

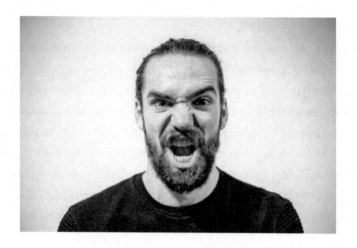

Figure 10.1 A very angry boss.

If this is a picture (Figure 10.1) of your boss waiting for you to arrive at work in the morning, you know that the day is not going to start well.

In many cases, however, it is not obvious. Have a look at the picture below.

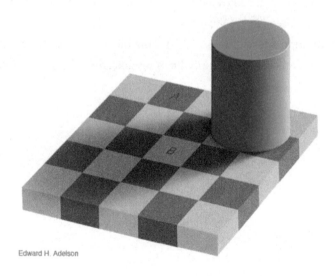

Edward H. Adelson

Figure 10.2 The chequerboard illusion

Figure 10.2 shows a chequerboard A green cylinder. A light source that shines from the right and casts a shadow across the chequerboard There are two

273

squares: one labelled "A" and a second labelled "B". Which of these squares is darker grey, square "A" or "B"[239]?

You might have guessed correctly. Indeed, there is no difference in colour! Flick to Appendix 8.1. for proof. Even if you know the answer, it is still very hard to convince yourself of this fact by looking at the figure once again. This figure demonstrates that biases shape the way we perceive our environment.

This chequerboard example also demonstrates that biases are often predictable. I had a strong suspicion about how your brain would interpret the image. "A" is the darker square. We might not understand in detail how the brain works, but nevertheless, I can anticipate your interpretation of the image. As biases are predictable, we can mitigate them through careful questioning.

Criticism of Thinking Fast and Slow

In *Gut Feelings*, Gigerenzer argues that decision-making models based on rules of thumb or heuristics do not necessarily lead to poor decision quality. Gigerenzer describes a technique that explains how humans can catch a ball that is flying through the air. All relevant information is captured in a single variable: the angle of gaze, which is the angle between the line from the eye to the ball and the second line from the eye to the horizon. The angle can be kept constant by adjusting the running speed (Figure 10.3). This illustrates that there is no need for complex mental mathematics. Simply keeping this angle fixed is sufficient.

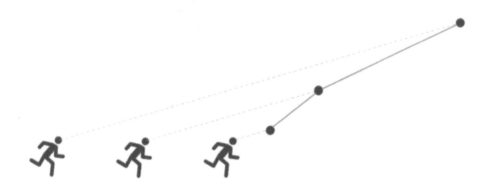

Figure 10.3. Fix your angle of gaze while running towards a ball. Reproduced from *Gut Feelings* by Gerd Gigerenzer.

---

[239] Adelson, 2005.

A constant stream of information arrives from the ball in the individual catching the ball. The person trying to catch the ball continuously updates the angle of gaze by moving around to keep the angle of gaze fixed. Other examples include the human ability to have meaningful conversations. When you have a conservation, you are constantly receiving information, visual and audio, which you use to plan and adjust the conversation.

The scenarios described above are fundamentally different from the experiments that Kahneman and Tversky conducted in the early 1970s[240]. All these experiments involved a single assessment of a probability, e.g., the Linda problem involves a short description followed by a single assessment.

It is a little awkward that this was known at the time. In 1967, Peterson and Beach published a study on statistical intuitions. Invoking the metaphor of the mind as an intuitive statistician, they concluded that 'probability theory and statistics can be used as the basis for psychological models that integrate and account for human performance in a wide range of inferential tasks'[241].

Creation of a judgement

Judgements do not pre-exist in the conscience of the human brain. Judgements are created once a question is asked. Knowledge and experience are used to construct a judgement.

An analogue of the creation of a judgement would be a pile of Lego® bricks that will be used to construct a toy car (Figure 10.4). The Lego® bricks represent the collection of memories and information you have available in your brain that are used to make a judgement.

---

[240] Kahneman & Tversky, 1973: Tversky & Kahneman, 1974.
[241] Lejarraga and Hertwig, 2021.

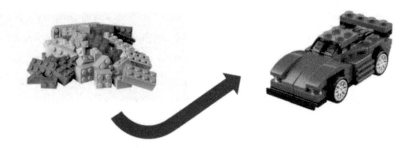

Figure 10.4. The analogy of a pile of Lego® bricks representing memories and information used by your brain to make a judgement of a Lego® car.

Biases, prejudices, favouritisms, prejudgements, and foregone conclusions are judgemental errors. These judgemental errors occur when mental shortcuts are used in the creation of a judgement. In the creation of a coherent worldview, the brain modifies knowledge and experiences. Biases occur subconsciously and affect our view of the world. Some Lego® bricks may be more easily accessible than others. Therefore, instead of a car constructed of blue and red bricks, a Lego® car might turn out red or blue (Figure 10.5).

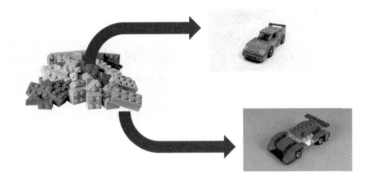

Figure 10.5. Biases result from the fact that some memories and information are more easily accessible by the brain than others. Hence, you might end up with a judgement of the red or blue car instead of the unbiased image of the Lego® that is multi-coloured.

Peterson, in his book *12 Rules for Life*, states: 'There is no complete and accurate story,' 'Only partial accounts and fragmentary viewpoints' and 'Memory is not an objective description of the past.'

Although it is straightforward to provide examples where System 1 fails, System 2 is also not infallible. For example, System 1 may have gathered accurate information, yet System 2 may process this information poorly and make a mistake. Conversely, System 1 may have gathered biased information and, therefore, despite System 2 processing it accurately, the conclusion may be incorrect due to a biased starting point. Systems 1 and 2 are complementary systems that work in tandem to produce more effective and efficient decision-making.

Another common misconception is the assumption that System 1 and System 2 occupy different areas of the brain. Kahneman[242] said, 'There is no part of the brain that either of the systems would call home.'

In conclusion:

> System 1 requires a small amount of cognitive resources, cannot be stopped voluntarily, and occurs unconsciously. However, there is an ongoing debate on the general applicability of these system 1-based decision models.
>
> System 2 requires a considerable amount of cognitive resources, can be stopped voluntarily, and occurs consciously.

Heuristic (rule-of-thumb) biases

[Difficulty: Red]

Awareness in itself does not mitigate bias. Knowing what causes bias allows for the design of elicitation methods that mitigate specific biases.

Five types of heuristic (rule-of-thumb) biases are particularly important.

> Anchoring: Overreliance on an initial piece of information
> Overconfidence: subjective confidence exceeds objective accuracy
> Availability bias: if something can be recalled easily, it must be important
> Causality of patterns: the human mind is a pattern-seeking device
> Base rate: appropriately adjusted base rate frequencies
> Survivorship bias: people systematically overestimate their chances of success

---

[242] Kahneman, 2011.

Anchoring

In a famous study, Dan Ariely, Drazen Prelec, and George Loewenstein[243] asked MIT students to bid on items in an auction. The researchers would hold up a bottle of wine, a textbook, or a cordless trackball and describe in detail how formidable it was. Then, each student had to write down the last two digits of their social security number first and their bid price second. Although the social security number has obviously nothing to do with their bid, the *anchoring* effect muddled the students' ability to judge the value of the items. Students with high social security digits paid up to 350% more than those with low digits. Students with numbers from 80 to 99 paid on average $26 for the trackball, while those with 00 to 19 paid around $9.

The participants in the MIT study were blissfully unaware that they were being anchored. Anchors can be as simple and seemingly innocuous as a comment offered by your spouse when you are rushing to get to work or a statistic appearing in the morning newspaper[244].

No one can eliminate the effect of anchoring; its impact is simply too widespread. However, there are techniques that can help reduce the influence of anchoring. Try to view the problem from different perspectives. Alternative starting points might yield different insights that could lead to a different judgement. Think about the problem before consulting others. The moment you learn about their idea, you are at risk of being anchored. Talk to as many people as possible. Actively seek different opinions. Be open-minded.

Anchoring can have a particularly strong impact when patients request a second opinion. When a doctor reviews the patient's files to create a second opinion, it is very hard to see how the first judgement made by the original medical team has no impact on the second judgement. I find it hard to believe that the first judgement does not anchor the second, and I question whether a second judgement can ever be truly independent.

Overconfidence

We systematically overestimate our knowledge and our ability to predict. *Overconfidence* can be measured by asking people to choose an upper and lower bound. In doing so, studies consistently found that the lower and upper bounds

---

[243] Ariely, Prelec, and Loewenstein, 2003.

[244] Hammond et al., 1999.

are too close together. Plous[245] said, 'No problem in judgement and decision-making is more prevalent and more potentially catastrophic than overconfidence.' Moore and Healy[246] found overconfidence to be the main factor that triggered wars, strikes, litigations, entrepreneurial failures, and stock market bubbles.

Few people are well calibrated. Rolf Dobelli[247] noted that 84% of Frenchmen estimate that they are above-average lovers, 93% of US drivers rated themselves as above-average in driving capabilities, 68% of the faculty rate themselves in the top-quartile for teaching abilities. All these assessments are affected by overconfidence bias. One study[248] reviewed 15,000 judgements on confidence intervals and concluded that participants were only accurate in their assessment 68% of the time[249].

People's first guesses often limit the range of possibilities that they consider[250]. Subject matter ability does not protect against overconfidence. Experienced researchers with a strong background in statistics are subjected to the same biases[251]. Experts suffer more from overconfidence than laypeople. Possibly because experts are expected to know their area of expertise.

How to reduce overconfidence

When someone is asked to identify an extreme value, the person being asked typically starts with a number that first comes to mind. As this number comes to mind first, it will be the most likely value in the person's judgement (Figure 10.6, top panel). After internalising this value. This value is gradually increased in steps until it becomes "extreme" in the perception of this person (Figure 10.6, middle panel). As soon as the value is perceived to be extreme, the person will stop increasing the value. This value is typically labelled as P90. However, a slightly higher number would be even more extreme simply because its value is higher. In fact, you just entered a whole range of values that are all "extreme"

---

[245] Plous, 1993.

[246] Plous, 2008.

[247] Dobelli, 2013.

[248] Lichtenstein et al., 1982.

[249] See *Are you well calibrated?* for details.

[250] Tversky and Kahneman, 1974.

[251] Tversky and Kahneman, 1971; Kahneman and Tversky, 1973.

but are nonetheless possible. Collectively, we refer to this set of values as the *Indifference range* (Figure 8.6, bottom panel). The indifference range terminate at the point where you enter values that are simply impossible, e.g., a probability that exceeds 100%.

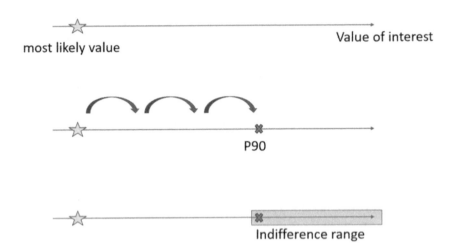

Figure 10.6. Typical thought process used to estimate extreme values. The upper panel shows the starting value; the middle panel shows how individuals progressively consider values that are increasingly unlikely, and the P90 is the point that they consider to be extreme. Following this process, you find yourself at the bottom end of the *Indifference range*, a set of values that are all considered extreme.

A fundamentally different approach is to start with the extreme values, P10 and P90, and make the final judgement of the median, aka the 50th percentage or P50, last[252] (Figure 10.7). One benefit of this approach is that when you start with very extreme, impossible, values, you enter the indifference range from the extreme lower end of the P10-indifference range or the extreme upper end of the P90-indifference range. When creating a judgement of extreme values, it is crucial to actively challenge these extreme estimates. Try hard to imagine scenarios that fall outside the range and adjust the extreme values accordingly.

Once you have defined the P10 and the P90, you can finally assess the P50 (Figure 10.7). One consideration when choosing a P50 is the shape of the probability distribution. Do you have any reasons to believe that the probability distribution should be skewed? Or is a symmetrical distribution more likely?

---

[252] Tversky and Kahneman, 1974; Hammond et al., 1999.

When I made my judgement on the length of my survival, I knew that the distribution was highly skewed. The P50 was much closer to the P10 than to the P90. Therefore, I chose my P50 accordingly.

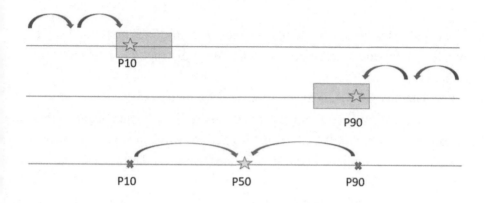

Figure 10.7. Sequence of assessment. Start with the extremes P10 and P90 and end with P50.

I recommend estimating the P10 and the P90 because more extreme P-values become increasingly difficult to judge. P10, P5, and P1 are all considered extreme values. Strict logic dictates that the probability increases for a value to fall into range between the P1 and the P99 is higher than the probability that a value falls in the range between the P10 and the P90; the range in the first case is 98% and this range decreased to 80% in the second case. Experiments failed to demonstrate this; the likelihood of a number falling into the range was observed to be constant as the width of the interval was decreased[253]. Thus one can draw the conclusion that humans are simply not very good at estimating extreme values – this observation strengthening our suggested approach.

The more extreme the percentage, the harder it is to make a correct judgement. P10 and P90 are on balance extreme values, but these values are not too extreme to estimate.

Despite the fact that I explained the process in great detail, some participants still did not follow the instructions I provided. For example, in one elicitation exercise I noticed that a participant had scribbled a number – a value that represented a most likely value – that consistently reappeared as a median

---

[253] Hora, 2007.

estimate. This median value was flanked by a lower and a higher estimate. So, this participant followed the process I warned against using (Figure 10.6).

How many kilometres did I cycle?

A couple of years ago, I had lunch with my family. That morning, I went on a two-hour bike ride. I posed the question, 'What distance had I cycled in these two hours?'

Our daughter gave an instant response: '12 kilometres.'

Well, I asked, 'What is the speed if you were walking?' Our daughter replied, '5 kilometres per hour.' Therefore, if I walked for two hours, I would cover 10 kilometres. We determined that walking speed was a good estimate of the lower bound.

To estimate the upper bound, I suggested 55 km/h. I asked my family how often they had seen a bike overtaken a car driving at 55 km/h. Not one of us had a recollection of a bike overtaking a car at that speed. Fifty-five kilometres per hour was deemed to be an appropriate estimate of the upper bond. Two hours at that speed makes for a total length of 110 km.

We established a reliable upper and lower estimate of 110 and 10 km, respectively. Now it was time to make an estimate of the median, P50.

After some discussion, my wife and the children decided that 60 km was the distance I had cycled. The true distance was 52 km.

This entire discussion over lunch took less than a minute. The final assessment was much more accurate than our daughter's blink-estimate of 12 km.

Are you well calibrated?

To assess how well someone is *calibrated*, a set of 10 questions has been developed. The answer is known for each question. For each calibration question, the participants were asked to provide a low (P10) and a high (P90) estimate, where:

P10 is the value for which the participant is 90% confident that the true value is *higher* than this particular value;

P90 is the value for which the participant is 90% confident that the true value is *lower* than this particular value.

There should be an 80% probability that the unknown value is captured in the range of values between P10 and P90. Or to put it in another way, 8 of 10 ranges should contain the true answer.

Before answering the question, ask yourself, 'Would I be shocked if the true answer was outside the interval I just defined?' If the answer is "yes", reconsider the extremes!

Here are 10 questions for you to consider:

What was the maximum wind speed at Heathrow Airport (London, UK) in 2020 (in km per hour)?

What is the population of Copenhagen, Denmark's capital?

What is the average ocean depth (in meters)?

What is the length of the Nile River (in km)?

What is the total number of medals won at the Tokyo 2020 Olympic Games?

What is the height of the Eiffel Tower (in meters)?

What is the probability that the main cause of a given person's death in the United States is heart disease?

What year was the first Nobel Prize awarded?

How many times was Merlin Streep nominated for an Academy Award?

What was the UK healthcare budget in 2020 (in billion UK pounds)?

Write the range as defined by the lower P10 and upper P90 estimates on a piece of paper. Now, look up the answers in the Appendix: Calibration questions.

Let me remind you that 8 of the 10 ranges should contain the true answer! I expect that even with the advanced warning to broaden the ranges, it is still likely that you have defined the P10–P90 interval too narrowly and that fewer than 8 of the ranges are sufficiently wide to capture the true answer.

Availability bias

The picture of the world we have created in our mind is based on images that come to mind most easily. However, this picture is not identical to the objective reality. Our worldview is biased due to the *availability bias*. Things do not happen more frequently just because we can dream them up more easily. The ease of recall, because it is rare and unusual, is not associated with the probability that the event would actually occur. John A. Paulus[254] wrote, 'remember that rarity in itself leads to publicity, making rare events appear commonplace', and Rolf Dobelli[255] said, 'We attach too much likelihood to spectacular flashy or loud outcomes. Anything silent or invisible is downgraded in our minds. We require other people's input to overcome the availability bias.

Human beings infer the chances of events from experience, which makes us overly influenced by dramatic events – those that leave a strong impression on our memory[256]. Although many people perish from common diseases such as heart attacks, organ failure, or asthma attacks, these events rarely make the headlines. This is opposed to shark attacks, car accidents, and war casualties. Each one of these events would make a headline!

The effect of availability bias is amplified by the fact that the typical human brain can track only seven facts at a time[257]. If humans had the capacity to hold let's say 200 facts in memory at once, the issue of availability bias would be greatly reduced.

After being diagnosed with cancer, I became much more aware of news items that feature cancer patients. They became more relevant to me personally. I will remember the stories told by Deborah James, Laura Nuttall, and Bill Turnbull for the rest of my life, simply because all three of them became victims of cancer. Do you remember their names and life stories? If not, it might well be because these individuals perished before you were diagnosed with your illness.

Lung cancer and coronary heart disease

Smoking causes lung cancer. This is not surprising. There is indeed a strong causal relationship between smoking and lung cancer. Mortality rates per 100,000 due to lung cancer are 329 for smokers and 13 for non-smokers. As a smoker, you are over 24 times more likely to die of lung cancer than a non-smoker.

---

[254] Paulus, 1988.

[255] Dobelli, 2013.

[256] Hammond et al., 1999.

[257] Miller, 1956.

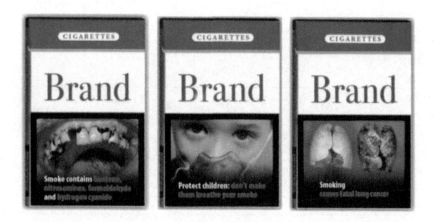

Figure 10.8. Three examples illustrating the effects of smoking.

Think about smoking for a moment. Your mind creates images of people sucking on a cigarette and inhaling the smoke deep into their lungs. Upon exhaling, the smoker is standing in the middle of a cloud of nasty-smelling fumes. Those of you who frequented cafés and bars in the 1990s will also remember that one had to wash all your clothes after an evening in town to get rid of the awful smoking smells. During my recent visit to Berlin, I entered several so-called *raucher* (smoker) cafés where people are still allowed to smoke, and I got flashbacks to the mid-1990s when I was living in Copenhagen. Back in those days smoking was still very normal thing to do. In addition, smoker's lungs make for vivid pictures as do pictures of innocent children who are breathing in second-hand smoke (Figure 10.8).

So, is lung cancer really the primary reason why people die from smoking?

Well, let's look at Table 10.1. This data is taken from the *Centers for Disease Control and Prevention* (CDC) site, which reports on the progress made over the past fifty years[258]. The *number to treat* to save one life is 304 for lung cancer and just short of 7 for coronary heart disease. Similarly, the absolute risk is much higher, 30.3, for coronary heart disease than for lung cancer.

---

[258] https://www.cdc.gov/tobacco/index.htm

	Lung cancer	Coronary heart disease
Smokers per 100,000	329	14,400
Non-smokers per 100,000	13	4,800
Relative risk per disease	$24 \left(= {}^{(329-13)}/_{13}\right)$	$2 \left(= {}^{(14,400-4,800)}/_{4,800}\right)$
Number to treat	$304.0 \left(= {}^{100,000}/_{329}\right)$	$6.94 \left(= {}^{100,000}/_{14,400}\right)$
Absolute risk per disease	$0.00316 \left(= {}^{(329-13)}/_{100,000}\right)$	$0.096 \left(= {}^{(14,400-4,800)}/_{100,000}\right)$
Absolute risk coronary heart disease versus lung cancer: 30.3 (=0.096/0.00316)		

Table 10.1. Difference between lung cancer and coronary heart disease.

Why is lung cancer strongly linked to smoking? In my humble opinion, it is mainly related to the fact that pictures of the black lungs of smokers and innocent children who breathe in second-hand smoke are much more persuasive than amputated limbs, mouths filled with tumours or blind eyes. Even the *CDC* website first lists lung cancer. Coronary heart disease follows on the second spot.

Causality of the patterns

Which of the following three sequences of heads-tails is most likely the result of a coin-flipping experiment using a fair coin (Figure 10.9)?

H-H-H-H-H-H

H-T-H-T-H-T

H-T-T-H-H-T

Figure 10.9. Six-coin tosses. H = Head, T = Tail.

I strongly suspect that most readers prefer the last sequence. This sequence appears to be generated using a random process because it lacks a clear pattern.

In fact, each sequence is equally likely! There are 64 equally likely combinations[259]. The human mind is a pattern-seeking device that infers that a pattern must exist. Tversky and Kahneman[260] referred to this fallacy as the *law*

---

[259] 0.5*0.5*0.5*0.5*0.5*0.5 = 1/64.

[260] Tversky and Kahneman, 1974.

of small numbers. The dataset is simply too small to make any definite conclusion on the underlying random process. The characterisation of the random process would require many more coin flips, i.e., deciding whether the coin is truly fair. The conclusion we draw based on a small set of samples is part of a larger issue of creating a view of the world that is simpler and more coherent than the data available justifies[261].

John A. Paulos wrote, 'People's inborn tendency to note coincidence and improbability, leading them to postulate connection and forces where there are none, where there is only coincidence.'

Correlation is not causation

Two variables are correlated if the high values of the two variables tend to coincide, i.e., large values of one variable tend to coincide with large values of a second variable. Likewise, small values also tend to coincide. Correlative relationships link two or more variables together, forming a possible connection Often, a correlation means absolutely nothing and is purely accidental[262].

Correlation does not imply *causation*. When interpreting correlations, just because two variables are correlated does not mean that a causal relationship exist. Causation implies that one variable directly influences or causes changes in another variable. To determine causation, additional evidence and rigorous research methods are typically required.

One possibility for the correlation without causation is the presence of an unobserved third factor. This third factor is controlling the two other variables and the correlation between these two variables is due to this missing variable. This is called a *spurious correlation*. Some methods can be used to spot spurious correlations:

Ensure that the sample is representative of the population;
Ensure that the dataset is sufficiently large to harness against the law of small numbers;

---

[261] Kahneman, 2011.

[262] https://www.statology.org/spurious-correlation-examples/ or https://tylervigen.com/spurious-correlations

Ensure that there is a strong p-value for the null hypothesis[263].

Blurred vision in Göttingen and placebo effect

On February 15, 2023, I was visiting friends in Göttingen. In the morning, I put in my contact lenses, but I struggled to focus. A blurred image appeared before my eyes. I removed my lenses and put them back in, but I still could not focus. I became worried about cancer growth in my brain. It is a well-known symptom that people's sight changes because of a growing tumour. Was this the first noticeable sign that my tumour was filling up my skull? A vivid mental image of inflating balloons appeared in my mind. A series of red, green, and blue balloons would appear at the base of my brain. As the balloon inflated, it gradually filled the entirety of my skull. I went back to the bathroom and swapped the contact lenses. Immediately, my vision became much clearer.

I am very aware that any changes I feel might be related to the progression of my disease. Any signs of deterioration would raise the question of whether the cancer growth has returned: a poor night's sleep or feeling a little light-headed or a slight headache or a rushing sound in my ears. This assessment is riddled with biases. To quote Kahneman, 'We are pattern seekers, believers in a coherent world, in which regularities appear not by accident.' The world in our heads is not a replica of reality but a simplified and polished version of the rough world we live in.

Two mechanisms are responsible for the illustrious placebo effect: belief and conditioning. In 1902, Ivan Pavlov began a series of classical experiments on conditioning. In his experiments, Pavlov demonstrated that the sound of a bell triggered salivation in dogs even before they were fed. Belief is the second mechanism. The belief that a drug, a procedure, or a caregiver will be effective might incline us towards a positive outcome. Dan Ariely, in his book *Predictable Irrational*, recounts when a nurse approached him with a syringe containing a painkiller and the relief he was experiencing prior to the actual injection of the painkiller. Dan's story is far from unique. Placebo effects are notoriously present in the treatment of pain[264].

---

[263] A p-value that is less than 5% is considered statistically significant. A p-value of 0.1% is statistically highly significant as in that case there is less than one in a thousand chance of being wrong.
[264] Colloca, 2018.

Because there are no pain receptors in the brain, patients with a brain tumour will not notice the moment seriously goes wrong inside their brains. John Gunter, in his book *Death be not Proud*, writes about a bruised apple. A rotting apple as a metaphor for a brain tumour is a powerful image; once the rotting process starts, the entire apple is affected within a single day. The solid texture of a fresh apple is replaced by a gooey brown substance with no coherent texture. How much brain-rot is required to notice a difference is still not clear to me. I struggle to see how patients with a brain tumour can experience a placebo effect.

...I was lucky. Six weeks later, I was told that there were no visible signs of cancer growth on my MRI scan.

Adjustment to the base rate

A judgement is an opinion that you have created after thinking carefully about a question. The starting point of any judgement is the base rate. In the absence of specific constraints, the base rate is the best estimate. In the era of internet search engines, many statistics can be found within minutes. These statistics will help you define a proper base rate for a specific judgement.

The adjustment of the base rate, or outside view, is what sets ordinary people apart from *super forecasters*[265]. A super forecaster can fine-tune his/her assessment to a single percentage point. This person actively seeks information that allows for small adjustments to the base rate. This fine tuning of the base rate leads to superior judgments.

Duke[266] shows in her book *How to Decide* a picture of a bison with a person and asks the reader to estimate the weight of the bison. According to Duke, 'I will be just guessing' is just a way to duck the answer, as this reply implies that anything less than perfect knowledge makes you answer random. However, even if you do not know the weight of the bison, there is a list of facts that we can confidently state:

A bison weighs more than a person;
You probably have an idea of the average weight of a cat or a dog;
You can judge the general size of the bison in relation to the surrounding cars and the man taunting it;

---

[265] Tetlock and Gardner, 2019.
[266] Duke, 2020.

You know how much you weigh;

You know that the bison weighs more than a man and;

You have some ideas of what cars weigh, and the weight of this car is probably greater than the weight of the bison.

You might not have perfect information on the weight of the bison, but you can certainly make a reasonable judgement. Writing down the list of facts will help you understand the gaps in your knowledge and find additional information.

The disadvantages of using probabilistic labels

One study[267] interviewed a panel of experts and recorded the wording they used to describe a certain feature and what they meant by these words in a probabilistic sense. The results of the study showed that the loose words used by the experts to describe their confidence are almost completely useless for any differentiation. Several terms such as *Hoped* and *Certain* covered the complete spectrum probabilities: from 0% to 100%.

Duke[268] reproduced the experiment and obtained much more accurate results. Duke proposed a two-step approach. In the first step, an assessment is made using labels that supply a description of probabilities. In the second step, these descriptions are translated into probabilities.

Personally, I would not follow this recommendation because these labels are inherently subjective and open to interpretation. Duke herself admits that "common terms are a blunt instrument" and that "using them comes at a steep price". Humans use the terms subjectively, and there is no common agreement on the probability associated with a specific term. I recommend using expert elicitation as a method to develop probabilistic estimates.

Survivorship bias: empty chairs in the hospital

June 2022, the oncology department in the hospital has a large waiting room with about 100 seats. A few seats are normally occupied by patients and carers who are waiting for an appointment for blood sampling, radiation treatment, or a doctor's appointment. Every time I walk past these seats, I wonder about the

---

[267] McLane et al., 2008.

[268] Duke, 2020.

chances of picking a random seat that is cancer-free. What is the chance to pick a single seat that is safe from cancer? The shocking reality for me is that of all these 100 seats, there are just two or three that are safe – cancer-free.

Apparently, over 95% of oncology patients believe that their chance of survival is better than that of their fellow patients. I believe that this is indeed the case. This is a prime example of *survivorship bias*. In Rolf Dobelli's book *The Art of Thinking Clearly,* survivorship bias is featured as the first bias. Rolf concludes the chapter as follows: '*Survivorship bias* means that people systematically overestimate their chances of success. Guard against it by frequently visiting the graves of once-promising projects, investments, and careers. It is a sad walk, but one that should clear your mind.'

I have often wondered how terminal patients can be free of bias and view the world in a truly objective way. Terminal patients who have an illness that will most likely result in their death. Patients who have been told that their life is likely to end within a given period. I have been lying awake in bed for hours with vivid images of dying patients. Not just any patient, it was me who was dying. Slowly losing the ability to do anything but sleep. There is also uncertainty about pain. Will there be a period of suffering? How long will it take for me to lose all my cognitive abilities? In such a state of mind, what does it take to be free of biases?

Motivational and heuristic (rule-of-thumb) biases

[Difficulty: Blue]

Two main types of bias exist: *motivational bias* and *heuristic (rule-of-thumb) bias.* Heuristic biases are the primary topic of the vast volume of psychological literature produced over the past decades. However, one should also be aware of motivational biases. Motivational biases affect people's judgement because they have an alternative motive, a hidden agenda, which favours a particular judgement.

Sir Ronald Aylmer Fisher argued that arguments should be "free from emotion" and "completely impartial". Yet, Fisher was on the payroll of an American tobacco firm. Hence, he did not approach the issue of smoking and cancer with the open mind that he championed as necessary in any good science. Fisher labels the claim that smoking might cause cancer as "propaganda", probably a "catastrophic and conspicuous howler" and a "frantic alarm" acting as the "Yellow Peril[269] of the modern time". Fisher was motivational biased.

Expert elicitation

[Difficulty: Green]

Expert elicitation is a process that aims to reduce the impact of biases and extract the most accurate and precise expert opinion. The word "elicitation" has its origin in the Latin word "elicio", which means "to draw out" or "to evoke".

Expert elicitation provides insight in situations where either there is very little data available or the data that is available is not representative for the uncertainty under investigation, i.e., the data does not help to place limits on the uncertainty. The process of expert elicitation is designed to force experts to reflect before they make a judgement.

Data book

I believe that the most effective way to reduce biases is to share all relevant data with the person making the judgement. The presentation of data in a clear and concise way will reduce the effect of:

Anchoring: all data are presented next to each other;
Overconfidence: the variability between different data points is useful for setting upper and lower estimates;
Causality of patterns: the data set as a whole will offer protection to spurious patterns;
Base rate: a comparison between the different data points is a good guide for estimating a base rate.

Balancing accuracy versus precision

Good judgements must be both *precise* and *accurate*. We can assess the quality of a set of judgements by comparing the judgements given to a set of questions with the known answers.

---

[269] The Yellow Peril is a racial colour metaphor that depicts the people of East and Southeast Asia as an existential danger to the Western world.

Table 10.2 shows the answers to 10 calibration questions provided by a participant to expert elicitation. All questions relate to probability; hence, only answers between 0% and 100% were possible. Most of the ranges defined cover nearly the complete interval of feasible solutions: 1%–100%. For example, question 5 has a P10 of 1%, a P50 of 50%, and a P90 of 100%. The expert who supplied these answers defined an extremely large interval and will achieve a high score for accuracy[270]. However, such judgement lacks precision and is therefore not informative. The amount of information conveyed in a judgement relates to the expert's ability to articulate that some values are more likely than others. If a judgement lacks precision, it is simply not helpful, as it does not provide the precision to differentiate between alternatives.

In the unlikely case that there is no information available, and the expert is indifferent what the value is most likely, one should use a uniform distribution[271]. All scenarios are equally likely. However, in a uniform distribution the P10 must be equal to 10%. Hence, we can conclude that a logical error has been made in all but one of the judgements (Table 10.2).

My interpretation of these judgements is that this individual tried to express complete ignorance and intentionally supplied estimates that do not contain any information. This is not helpful; we might as well have used a die or flipped a coin.

	Q1	Q2	Q3	Q4	Q5	Q6	Q7	Q8	Q9	Q10
P10	0.05	0.02	0.1	0.005	0.01	0.01	0.01	0.01	0.01	0.01
P50	0.3	0.3	0.7	0.01	0.5	0.2	0.1	0.7	0.1	0.4
P90	1	1	1	0.1	1	1	1	1	1	1

Table 10.2. Lack of precision. These answers are non-informative because these probability estimates cover the full range of possible solutions.

---

[270] An expert who sets a P10 probability at 0% and a P90 probability at 100% will receive a high score for accuracy.

[271] A uniform distribution has an assigned equal probability for all possible outcomes. A uniform distribution is a straight horizontal line.

At the other extreme end, we have the answers provided by a second participant. This expert supplied highly informative narrow intervals (Table 10.3). For example, the answers to question 2, a P10 of 1% and a P90 of 5%, made up a mere 4% interval. However, after a comparison between the provided intervals and the known answers, it became clear that only one ranges supplied contained the true answer.

	Q1	Q2	Q3	Q4	Q5	Q6	Q7	Q8	Q9	Q10
P10	0.04	0.01	0.4	0.01	0.2	0.02	0.02	0.15	0.01	0.4
P50	0.07	0.02	0.7	0.02	0.35	0.04	0.04	0.2	0.03	0.45
P90	0.12	0.05	0.95	0.05	0.6	0.1	0.07	0.4	0.08	0.5

Table 10.3. Lack of accuracy. These answers are inaccurate, as none of these ranges has a known answer.

Having worked with experts over many years, I realise how difficult it is to provide a clear set of instructions. Therefore, just to re-iterate, the lack of accuracy is a result of the overconfidence bias. The advice I give to experts is that they should aim to set the lower bound at a value that they can defend, i.e., the expert should ask themselves whether there is a feasible scenario in which the value provided could be true. However, this value should be surprising to the expert. The other extreme, lack of precision, has more to do with the desire to dodge the question. I suspect that these participants struggle with making informed judgements or educated guesses. It is extremely rare that judgments are made in the complete absence of any data or experience. Experts might not realise that in most judgements are educated guesses. However, there is inherent value in being a little less wrong and a little closer to right[272].

---

[272] Duke, 2020.

Fast and frugal trees

[Difficulty: Blue]

An expert is somebody who has a broad and deep understanding and competence in terms of knowledge, skill, and experience through practice and education in a particular field. A doctor is an expert. As a doctor gains experience, (s)he will develop heuristic models. A heuristic model is a set of rules. Like 'I will prescribe an antibiotic if the patient in front of me has a higher fever (>39 degrees Celsius) and has a productive cough.'

In 2018, Gerd Gigerenzer gave a presentation titled *The Heuristics Revolution*. Gigerenzer advocated simple decision models based on rules of thumb. These simple models enable experts to use their intuition in their decision-making process. Gigerenzer made a set of predictions based on a rule-of-thumb model, *Fast and Frugal Trees*, which was more accurate than a second set of predictions based on a more complex regression analysis[273]. These Fast and Frugal Trees consist of three to five questions with simple binary Yes-No answers[274]. Given its simplicity, this method is attractive for resource-constrained tasks.

Although most rules of thumb will be very useful in quick decision making, there will be situations where such rules of thumb do not work. These rules of thumb form a *mental model* that filters out any conflicting observations. The removal of certain observations creates a bias that might prevent continuous learning and hinder the improvement of your skills as a decision maker. Thus, gaining experience is not always helpful when experts hone their decision-making skills. To quote the Danish scientist and Nobel laureate Niels Bohr, 'An expert is a person who has made every possible mistake within his or her field.'

Concluding remarks: Human judgement

The two different ways of developing a judgement are simply labelled System 1 and System 2. System 1 is the default mode and requires a small

---

[273] These results were published in 2007 in *Gut Feelings*. Given the progress made in AI and machine learning since the book was published, it would be very interesting to rerun the experiment.

[274] The Fast and Frugal Tree is the equivalent of a classification tree in machine learning. In a classification tree, choices are made to ensure that the threshold values are optimally chosen and the most predictive attributes are selected.

amount of cognitive resources. System 1 simplifies reality by creating believable stories. System 2 requires a considerable amount of cognitive resources and system 2 thinking is our method to create rational judgements.

Understanding the interplay between these two systems helps us navigate everyday decisions. Becoming aware of this interplay empowers us to make better-informed decisions.

We have almost reached the end of our journey together. There is one chapter left that will conclude our journey and my book. Let us finish the book on an optimistic, more positive note!

Appendix: Proof of visual illusion

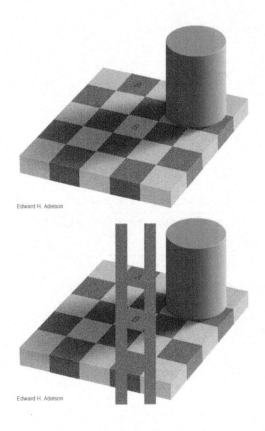

Figure A.10.1. Proof that squares A and B have the same grey shading[275]. Even if you know the answer, it is still difficult, impossible, to convince yourself that squares A and B have the same grey colour.

---

[275] Adelson, 2005.

Appendix: Calibration questions

Answers to the calibration questions:

Question:	Answer:
What was the maximum wind speed at Heathrow airport (London, UK) in 2020 (in km /h)?	96 km/hr
What is the population of Copenhagen, Denmark's capital?	1.4 million
What is the average ocean depth; in meters?	3,682 m
What is the length of the river Nile in kilometres?	6,650 km
What is the total number of medals won at the Tokyo 2020 Olympic Games?	1,080 medals
What is the height of the Eiffel Tower; in meters?	324 m
What is the probability that the cause of death is heart disease in the US?	25%
What was the year in which the first Nobel Prize was awarded?	1901
How many times was Merlin Streep nominated for an Academy Award?	21 times
What was the UK healthcare budget in 2020 (in billion UK pounds)?	269 billion pounds

Part 4

Afterword

'After my expectation had been reduced to zero, every day became a bonus and I began to appreciate everything I had. While there is life, there is hope. Be brave, curious, determined, and overcome the odds. It can be done.'

Stephen Hawking in *Brief Answers to Big Questions*

'This book carries the urgency of racing against time, of having important things to say. Paul confronted death – examined it, wrestled with it, accepted it – as a physician and patient. Although the last few years have been wrenching and difficult – sometimes impossible – they have also been the most beautiful and profound of my life.'

Lucy Kalanithi in the epilogue of Paul's book *When Breath Becomes Air*

'Remembering that I'll be dead soon is the most important tool I've ever encountered to help me make the big choices in life.'

Steve Jobs

Abstract Afterword

I decided to be an optimist. An optimist can also be a realist. I know that the odds of surviving the first two years after my brain surgery are very small indeed. Combining an optimistic life attitude with a very dire outlook on the future has been the hardest thing I have been struggling with since my diagnosis in early June 2022.

I am very grateful that I was alive long enough to finish this book. This makes me feel jubilant. I got so much pleasure from writing.

I believe we should focus on the here and now. We all live in the moment. We must focus on the decisions, the choices we can make. We all must choose what activities we pursue in our finite life and how we will spend our time in this incredible place we can call home.

Infinite happiness

I would like you to participate in this thought experiment. Just imagine that you have a 50% chance to survive another day. This additional day gave you much enjoyment. You realise that your enjoyment would double if you could live another day, day 2. However, the chance of living on this second day would be 25% (=50% * 50%). Each day going forward, your enjoyment would double and the chance of living that day would halve.

How much personal happiness would be created in such a world?

The game described above is better known as St. Petersburg paradox. This problem was first proposed by Daniel Bernoulli in 1738[276]. The incremental happiness doubles each day, and the chance that this event materialises halves each day. Let us calculate our expected value for this thought experiment. We have a 50% chance of gaining incremental happiness of 2 on the first day[277]. On the second day, the chance is halved to 25%, but the incremental happiness is doubled to 4. This process of halving the chances and doubling happiness continues each day until eternity. The expected happiness of this thought experiment is $\left(\frac{1}{2}\right)2 + \left(\frac{1}{4}\right)4 + \left(\frac{1}{8}\right)8 + \cdots$, or $\sum_{k=1}^{\infty} \left(\frac{1}{2^k}\right)\left(2^k\right) = 1 + 1 + 1 + 1 + \cdots = \infty$. You gain infinite happiness in this game!

For nearly 300 years, the sharpest mathematical minds have not been able to solve this puzzle. Perhaps the solution to this paradox is completely obvious; no life is infinite in duration[278].

Pluk de dag (Living in the moment)

There is a Dutch expression: '*Pluk de dag.*' Which literally translates as "Pick the day" but I would translate its meaning as "*Living in the moment*". Although these three words in Dutch and four words in English are very short

---

[276] In the original version of St. Petersburg paradox Bernoulli proposes a coin flip game in which one flips until the coin land on the tail.

[277] The "2" has been chosen rather arbitrary, but this choice will make the mathematics somewhat easier, as will become clear in a moment.

[278] Or one could apply a concave utility function...

sentences, it will take some more words to properly explain this concept – *Carpe diem* or *Living in the moment.*

I have been writing about my bike rides. I have been riding my bike three times a week, and in each bike ride, I cover a distance of fifty to sixty kilometres in a little over two hours. Upon leaving the house, I have fifty-five kilometres to cover – there is no point in rationalising how I will experience these two hours. There are simply too many hills to climb, wind gusts, and potholes to consider. I know about a pothole located in a bend in the road just south of Lawshall, but this fact is simply not relevant to me for now – at this point in time – as it takes me over an hour to get to this pothole. Likewise, the climb out of the village is no longer relevant once I have reached the top of the hill. What is important is how I feel in the here and now. How easy is it to push the pedal down? Should I stand up from the saddle to push the pedal with some extra force? Are there any potholes to consider just in front of the bike? Is this gush of wind a precursor to a prolonged windy period?

There is a second analogue activity that I can use to illustrate the concept of *Living in the Moment,* and that activity is walking. Apart from the obvious parallels to cycling – there is no point in anticipating the entire walk at the time you start your walk – the walking activity enables me to have some delightful experiences. Observing the bright red rose hips, the deep purple sloe berries, and the yellow leaves in late afternoon sunlight. The wind rustling the leaves and the smell of autumn dampness. Walking is a slow process; therefore, a walker needs a certain degree of patience. I am not sure how our teenagers will cope with walking in thirty-forty years' time when they will be my age – in their early fifties. Will the next generation have the patience to slow down and take it all in?

Personally, I find walking is a very effective way to slow down, to create a clear mind, and spend time reflecting and thinking. I am not the only person who has this experience. Oliver Burkeman, in his book *Four Thousand Weeks*, describes a walk he has done many times in the Yorkshire Dales. Burkeman states: '…all I am doing is walking, a skill which I haven't appreciably improved since around the age of four…'

I did not always have this philosophy of life. As a matter of fact, this – Living in the moment – life attitude was very much forced upon me. I have spent most of my life on a three- to four-year rolling planning horizon. The reason for me to adopt this "three-to-four-year planning horizon"-life's attitude is based on quantum physics and chaos theory.

In 1927, Werner Heisenberg published a thesis that is generally referred to as the Uncertainty Principle. Heisenberg demonstrated that one cannot accurately measure the position and speed of a particle. The more accurately you measure the speed of a particle, the less precise is the measurement of the location of the particle. The reverse also holds. If you can measure the location of a particle, its speed will remain unknown. Although even Einstein struggled with his acceptance of this theory with his famous quote 'God does not play dice,' many subsequent studies have demonstrated that at a fundamental level this is how the universe works[279]. The universe is inherently uncertain and gone are the days when we believed that if we could only learn the state of all particles, we would be able to make a perfect prediction of the future.

In *The Essence of Chaos*, Edward Lorenz described the scenario of how 'The flap of a butterfly's wing in Brazil can set off a tornado in Texas.' Edward was working as a meteorologist when he noticed that the model, he developed gave non-reproducible results. The second calculation run gave a very different answer than the first. The culprit was a small difference in the rounding error in the barometric pressure readings 29.5168 was rounded to 29.517, a value difference of less than 0.0007%. It did not take long before Lorenz realised the cause of the problem. Many of the relationships in the model developed by Lorenz were non-linear, they were exponential. Therefore, multiplying a number that is slightly different many times over will result in a solution that will be completely different. Weather is a classic example of a dynamic system, the equations used to model the flow of gases and fluids in the atmosphere are all exponential relationships. Because of these exponential relationships, the results of the model are prone to be affected by slight differences in the starting conditions. We are simply not able to measure our environment with a sufficient degree of precision. Tomorrow's weather predictions might be useful in your decision whether or not to take your umbrella with you. However, if you want a useful prediction concerning the weather four weeks you might as well get yourself one of these famous dart-throwing chimpanzees. The mathematics of the problem – the exponential relationships between the variables and our inability to measure precise initial conditions – simply prevents us from predicting the future. This logic is true for weather forecasting, as well as

---

[279] Stephen Hawking, 2018.

forecasting in general. We simply are not able to predict what the future has in store for us four years.

How do you prepare yourself for the future?

I realised in my early thirties that randomness prevents us from making useful predictions of a distinct future. Therefore, I tried to optimise those decisions that would determine my happiness over the coming months and two years. Those events that materialised next month were much more important than those that would happen two years into the future. Events that might happen in a decade that I considered too uncertain to even seriously think about. I saved a lot of mental energy by ignoring the possible impact of these long-term events.

I also realised that you must repeatedly update your anticipated future. I made a conscious decision to ensure that I allocated time in my busy life to assess where my life was going, whether I was still happy, and whether whatever I was doing would lead to future opportunities. I made a reassessment of my situation each time I faced a choice that was sufficiently important to me and my family. I anticipated the advice given by Brother David Steindl-Rast in his inspirational video *Want to be Happy? Be Grateful*: Stop, look, and go.

Ask yourself what is important to you right now.

And guess what – whatever your answer is to this question – it will be different had I asked your younger self a decade ago. As we mature, our priorities change. For example, after I started my Ph. D. in geology, geology was the single most important factor in my life. A decade later, I finished my Ph. D. and became a doctor in geology. At that point, my wife and I were thinking about starting a family. Therefore, we gave up our city lifestyle and our apartment in central Copenhagen and we moved to the outskirts of the city. We exchanged our Peugeot GTI for a much larger and much slower family car. Our value system – the things that were important to us – had changed.

Life is like sailing. You must decide when to tack. Change direction – turning through the wind – and find a new course. The moment you decide to change direction, you must be fully committed. This way of life is not for the faint hearted. Any sailors amongst you will have experienced the flapping sails and pulling of the ropes as the boat finds a new direction.

I don't know which life philosophy has my preference. My preference may simply be irrelevant. I might not have a choice in the matter as I probably will not be around in five to ten years to accommodate these long-term plans. I am afraid that my days of plain sailing are gone forever. For now, I am living my life in the now. I am a cyclist and walker.

Flow

Humans have a lifespan of about *Four Thousand Weeks* according to Oliver Burkeman[280]. Limited time is not the fundamental problem. Burkeman states '…[we] feel pressured to live by a troublesome set of ideas about how to use our limited time…' I strongly suspect that these "troublesome set of ideas" that Burkeman was talking about were not Csikszentmihalyi's[281] "positive aspects of human experiences". Csikszentmihalyi begins his book *Flow* with the following: 'The positive aspects of human experiences – joy, creativity, the process of total involvement with life' and 'a joyful life is an individual creation that cannot be copied from a recipe.'

Abraham Maslow[282] published a paper titled *A Theory of Human Motivation* in which he defined a hierarchy of needs. The hierarchy of needs is one of the best-known physiological theories of motivation, i.e., what makes people happy. This hierarchy suggests that people are motivated to fulfil basic needs (food, water, and air) before moving on to other, more advanced needs. The highest level is what Maslow defined as "self-actualisation" – self-fulfilment through pursuit of moral ideals and creativity for their own sake.

Tom and David Kelley wrote in their book *Creative Confidence* that 'a *calling* is a sense that you are contributing to a higher value or to something bigger than yourself' and 'you should be able to feel passion, purpose and meaning in whatever you do.'

Many of these ideas were known to the Ancient Greeks, as Epicurus stated: 'one can only be happy and free from suffering by living wisely, soberly and morally' and 'a person who is kind and just to others will have no fear.'

Paul Kalanithi wrote in *When Breath Becomes Air*: 'Death comes for all of us. It is our fate as living, breathing, and metabolising organisms. Part of the cruelty of cancer, though, is not that it limits your time; it also limits your energy, vastly reducing the amount you can squeeze into a day. Severe illness was not life-altering, it was life-shattering. Death may be a one-time event, but living

---

[280] Burkeman, 2021.

[281] Csikszentmihalyi, 1990.

[282] Abraham, 1943.

with terminal illness is a process. It felt less like an epiphany – a piercing burst of light, illuminating What Really Matters and more like someone had just firebombed the path forward.'

Keeney[283] wrote in *Value Focussed Thinking*: 'Over the years, I have spent considerable effort thinking about and writing down my strategic objectives for my life. This effort has been worthwhile because I have repeatedly invoked these objectives in my decision-making. [These objectives] define both who I am, in that they have guided my past and who I want to be, in that they indicate where I want to go.'

I decided in April 2022 to write a book. Reflecting on this period, I am not even sure whether I had a choice – it felt to me that I simply had to complete a book about this maelstrom of emotions that I was subject to. I was never sure whether I had enough time to finish writing any of my stories.

The book *Flow* by Csikszentmihalyi made a deep impression on me. When in "flow" you enter a creative state, you lose track of time and become completely immersed in an activity for its own sake. The book motivated me and gave me the strength to continue my writing journey. Fyodor Dostoyevsky wrote in *The Brothers Karamazov*, 'The mystery of human existence lies not in just staying alive, but in finding something to live for.'

I am very grateful that I have been given the opportunity to write in good health. This makes me happy. 'It is not happiness that makes us grateful, but gratefulness that makes us happy!' to quote Brother David Steindl-Rast[284].

Brother David Steindl-Rast told his audience a story about himself spending some time in Afrika, where there was no access to clean drinking water, and how he struggled to get hold of water suitable for consumption. Upon his return to Austria, Brother David decided to label the mains waterpipe to remind him every day to be grateful for having access to clean water.

A year after my operation, my life has returned to normal. Although this is not the old normal, it is the new normal. I am very conscious about the fact that one day I will simply forget to be grateful, grateful to live another day, grateful to open my eyes in the morning, and grateful to spend another day with my family. I hope and wish that gratefulness has become an intrinsic part of my life.

---

[283] Keeney, 1993.

[284] https://www.ted.com/talks/david_steindl_rast_want_to_be_happy_be_grateful?language=en

I am an atheist. I do not believe that there is anything after death. Gratefulness as a constant reminder is parallel to praying. Like praying, I will take a break once a day to reflect on my life and be grateful for it.

Letters to an old friend

I met my friend in Copenhagen, Denmark, about 25 years ago. Both of us were in our early thirties, and we shared many beers together. We lost touch when I left academia. After I came to grips with the knowledge that I had a brain tumour I wrote the following letter to my friend:

5 December 2022, Suffolk

Dear Friend,

I woke up around 6:45 this morning. The clicking sound of the expanding central heating pipes may have been the cause of my early awakening. It is winter, and the heating is set to come on in the morning for an hour. I was lying in bed in the dark. I heard our son[285] in the house – presumably, he was getting up and getting his breakfast sorted. I also heard the sleeping sounds made by my wife, who was lying next to me in bed. Six months previously, I was lying in the same spot at the same time, having already been awake for several hours. During that period, I woke up very early each morning. The combination of the shock that I lost 25 years of my life and the side effects of the steroids I was taking at that time was sufficient to wake me up early in the morning – each and every morning. I still cannot get my head around the fact that I had a brain tumour the size of a golf ball, which I simply did not notice. During the operation, the tumour was removed and the hole that was left behind has been shrinking ever since. There has not been any sign yet that the cancer is growing. So, for now, I am progression free.

Over the past six months, my life has returned to normal. "Normal" is not normal for normal people. I have about twelve months left of the sixteen months I was given at the time of diagnosis. In 2019, an article appeared in Scientific American that described glioblastoma, the cancer I have been diagnosed with, as "The most common form of malignant brain cancer – called a glioblastoma – is notoriously wily and considered the deadliest human cancers".

---

[285] I have removed the names for confidentiality reasons.

I have not shared this quote with my family. I know that my wife knows. Both my children are in denial of the seriousness of the situation. Although both children know that I had a tumour in my brain, neither my wife nor I have shared the prognosis. The "16-month"-bit. This has been the hardest thing for me to deal with; not telling the children all the facts, holding back the full story, and leaving out this crucial detail. I remember discussing the survival data with one of my colleagues five months ago. A close colleague of mine, who happens to be a statistician, told me that I would be dead in two years. I did not reply because I knew that he was very likely to be right. He wrote to me an email about a month later after the conversation that 'I should carefully listen to my oncologist on my way to recovery.' As I am alive today, I might also be alive two, four, or ten years. This was my rationale for going back to work. I needed the structure of a day's work. A reason to get out of bed in the morning.

I returned to work in September. I started my job as part of a small team of Decision Scientists. Six years later, I am the only Decision Scientist left in the company. This morning, I sat down behind my desk and went through my inbox and found an email that a collaborator had sent on Saturday morning. I had been awarded a Catalyze award. Catalyze awards are part of the company incentive scheme that enables colleagues to recognise each other. I followed the link and read:

Ioannis Psallidas awarded **You**

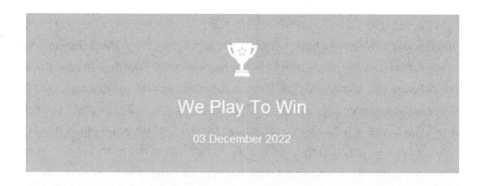

We Play To Win

03 December 2022

REAL forum presentation

Thank you very much for the REAL forum presentation for Protocol complexity. You spent time drafting slides, rehearsing your part, and preparing for the REAL forum. Your presentation was top notch and you delivered the messages in a clear, professional and concise way. I was impressed that we delivered the talk on time and with the number of colleagues attending the forum. We manage to break the record of attendance in this forum and this is because of your hard work and delivery. Many thanks for your time and effort. One of the greatest teams that I have ever worked with and such a motivated group of people to deliver tools and framework that will accelerate our pipeline. I am so happy working together on the protocol complexity tool. Best wishes, Ioannis

I promptly pressed the reply button and responded as follows:

> *You are completely right: this was one of the, if not the, BEST project I worked on in my entire career! I wonder what we need to do to exceed this achievement in 2023.*
> *Despite the small hiccup during the spring/summer we had a blast!*
> *Cheers Bart*

After sending more emails, I had a call with one of my Swedish colleagues. I wanted to talk to one of my colleagues about elicitation modeling. Although I planned the meeting for 30 minutes, we ended up talking for almost 50 minutes – it is not unusual for us to run over time in our lively debates where we are trying to set the world right. Both of us are fascinated by expert elicitation (i.e., a structured conversation with experts) and simple role-of-thumb models. These simple models tend to outperform very sophisticated machine learning models when making predictions in an uncertain world.

Over the past six months, I have spent most of my time writing. I have written three books in parallel: an autobiography, a diary, and a third book that I refer to as Bart's Insight[286]. The latter requires some explanation. Over the past 25 years, I have been working as a Decision Analyst. In this period, I have done much thinking about the topic of decision analysis, I have read a lot about different ways of building statistical models, and I have explored different techniques to interact with experts.

Writing a book was on my bucket list for over a decade, but I simply could not find a suitable topic. That changed six months ago. The starting point was that I wanted to write a text that is easy to read, a text with no jargon or complex sentences. I am well on the way now. I have written well over 80.000 words. I would like to have a first draft readily between Christmas 2022 and the New Year.

A couple of days ago, I had an appointment with the MRI scanning team. This was my fourth MRI scan. My fifth scan, if I include the CT scan. The image of the CT scan showed the first indication that something was seriously wrong with me – this was the image that put my life upside down. Magnetic resonance imaging (MRI) is a type of scan that uses strong magnetic fields and radio waves to produce detailed images of the inside of the human body. An MRI scanner is a very noisy machine. Patients are provided with ear plugs before they enter the large tube at the centre of the scanning machine. The volume of clicking and humming sounds made by the MRI machine is deafening.

I am not allowed to drive because of the risk of seizures while driving. Therefore, my wife dropped me off at the MRI scanner located in the hospital before she went shopping for a rucksack for our son, who is going on an expedition to Norway this summer. He does not appear to be engaged in the slightest, but I do wonder whether he is tricking us all. He is going to kayak, camp, hike, and fish. All the activities 14-year-old boys love to do…unless he is truly not engaged…

My wife went out to purchase some typical British treats for my parents and my brother's family. This weekend my brother and his family are coming over to visit us. They will take the ferry on Thursday night and arrive Friday morning at

---

[286] This is the book you are currently reading.

our place. They will stay with us for the weekend and return Sunday evening. My brother has twins – a daughter and a son.

I have asked my brother to bring along old, warm clothes because there is a large stack of wood lying in the back of the garden that must be moved into the woodshed. There is also a massive pile of branches that we can burn if we have a couple of spare hours. We also have two Christmas trees that are currently standing in a bucket of water outside. The plan is to decorate these trees over the weekend with the help of my niece. My niece loves Christmas! It is winter, and the temperature will drop below freezing over the coming days, so I hope it is not going to be too cold.

Over the summer, we bought our son a motorbike. A "pit bike". He has been riding in our garden for hours at end – the same loop over and over again. A couple of weeks ago, I decided to clean his bike; also, rather unusually, he had not been riding it for a week. After some prodding from my side, it turned out that he could not start the bike. I cleaned the carburettor, chain and air filter. Put it all back together and asked our son to start the engine. It worked! As a finishing touch, I tweaked the screw in the carburettor to increase the revs and make it run more smoothly. This all sounds like fun, but it is no fun when you are dealing with a grumpy teenager. It is a test of patience. However, I got some comfort from a village friend who picked our son up from school in his soft-top car. My friend asked him about his pit bike; apparently, he had been paying close attention during the bike maintenance session!

I spoke to our daughter a couple of days ago. She is nineteen now. Second year at the university We spoke about her coming around for Christmas, and I asked her whether she had wrapped her present and finished her poem. The poem is of critical importance – the basic idea behind the poem is to make fun of the person you bought a present for.

Today, it is 5 December; Sinterklaas. Sinterklaas is a Dutch tradition that goes back centuries. The story goes that Sinterklaas is coming from Spain each year on his steamship. His helpers are called "Zwarte Pieten". Pieten are black because of the soot they scrape off the inside of the chimney while they descend the chimney. In the past few years, much fuss has surrounded the Zwarte Pieten. There was a heated discussion regarding the origin of the concept of Zwarte Pieten, and it was suggested that Zwarte Pieten originated from slaves. Thanks to a few disgruntled people, we now have an annual Zwarte Pieten debate that tends to be very heated!

One of the Sinterklaas traditions is to give each other a chocolate letter. It did require a little planning, but we managed to get four letters. The chocolate letter is the first letter of our name. One we posted to the address where our daughter is living, and the three others are lying on the coffee table downstairs.

I am forever grateful that you insisted that I ask my wife to marry me. I cannot remember whether we were in a pub or in the argon lab (in my judgement both options are equally likely!) but I do remember that your statement made a real impression on me. A couple of months later, I called my future father-in-law to ask for his daughter's hand.

A few years later, when you and your wife visited my wife and me at our house in Bagsværd. The four of us were sitting in our kitchen, and your wife had just announced that she was pregnant. I remember the look of sheer horror on your face when our daughter was sick. My wife and I were clearing up the mess as if nothing had happened. Events like that were happening frequently at that time.

As I wrote to you in my previous email, I feel great now, but the fact that I have been fine over the past six months is no guarantee for the coming six months. In my judgement I have about six months left to live once the tumour returns.

It is almost 21:00 pm now, so it is time for me to join my wife in the living room downstairs and watch some telly!

Cheers Bart

Six months later, I decided to write a second letter to my dear old friend:

August 1, 2023, Suffolk

Dear Friend,

On July 4, 2023, I saw my doctor appointment to discuss the MRI scan that was made in the previous week. My wife and I arrived at a very busy hospital site with fifteen minutes to spare. We were stuck in stationary traffic, so I got out of the car and walked toward the outpatient department. I felt stressed and went to the toilet to get some relief. After I washed my hands and put on a face mask, I walked to the oncology department. During the previous meetings with the doctor, I was joined by my wife. This time, I was myself.

My doctor told me that a small cancer growth could be seen on the scan. He switched on the computer and viewed the black and white image of the MRI scan. A white speck with a diameter of approximately 7 mm revealed the location of the cancer tumour. I left the room in a state of shock – I was feeling lightheaded. I eventually met my wife in the corridor. I broke the news to her, and we decided to have a coffee at the hospital restaurant. I told her the details of the MRI scan results and that "there are lots of options available to me". Knowing full well that all these options are far less effective than the TMZ I that had been taken previously.

When I visited my parents in June 2023, I expressed my hope. What I meant by being "hopeful" was that I judged the likelihood of being alive at Christmas to be about 40%, i.e., I had a proper decent shot to reach Christmas. Before the tumour-free MRI scan in March 2023, I was convinced that I would not be alive on Christmas Day 2023. Now I am no longer a progression-free survivor; the tumour was regrowing inside my skull. Looking back, I am surprised that I survived almost a year being "progression free". I always knew that the chances of surviving a glioblastoma were very small indeed. This might sound very weird, but I was almost relieved. Knowing that the tumour has returned makes me feel even more determined to make the most of our trip to Tanzania. My wife asked me whilst we were driving home after the hospital visit whether I still wanted to go ahead with our trip. It struck me as a stupid question.

When we spoke to my doctor the next day, he advised against our planned holiday. We promised him to take some steroid tablets with us for me to take before our flights, and my wife pointed out the presence of nearby hospitals. He realised that we had made up our minds and gave us his WhatsApp contact number.

I woke up at 5:30 am because of rain falling on the Velux bedroom window. I realised it was Monday morning in wet and rainy England. I was lying again in my own bed after a hiatus of sixteen days. We just returned from our Tanzanian holiday. Tanzania is fantastic. The animals, the people, the food, the smells, the sounds, and the colours really made this the holiday of a lifetime[287].

---

[287] We spent the first week on safari and visited three national parks (Lake Manyara, Ngorongoro Crater and Serengeti). We literally took thousands of pictures of elephants, lions, leopards, cheetahs, rhinos (from very far away – so you a dark dot in the distance is the only photographic evidence), giraffes, zebras, various types of gazelles, hippos, crocks, ostriches, and numerous very colourful birds. Our local guide, Pilagio, was

Given my illness, there is a very high likelihood that this trip was indeed my last visit to another continent. It was almost certainly the last family holiday with all four of us[288].

This final trip was of great importance to me as I regarded it as my final attempt to excite our children. Ensure they appreciate the beauty of nature. We live in nature – we depend on nature. Animals, flowers, and the sky filled with stars are all part of nature[289].

---

fantastic. He did his utmost to make us feel comfortable and had a real sense of humour. Although we had to get up early in the morning to get ready for our morning game drive, the children did not once complain! During the week, I sensed a deep connection developed between the children and Pilagio. I was very pleased by this! In the Serengeti, we had an early morning hot air balloon trip. We drifted for about an hour over the treetops, spotting animals and watching the sunrise. The trip ended with a bumpy landing. It took several attempts to finally put down the hot air balloon. The accommodation was superb – each place we stayed in was unique and the food was excellent – without exception.

The second week we spent in Zanzibar. Zanzibar is an island, known as Unguja by the locals, off Tanzania's coast. After a couple of days exploring Stone Town, the historical part of Zanzibar. Stone Town is a true maze – I was lost the moment I stepped outside the hotel. I went for several wanders and became completely disorientated every single time. Only when you leave the narrow alleyways and enter the wider streets that surround the old city centre can you find your way back. We were fortunate that our hotel was part of an old palace, which was relatively easy to find on the map.

We ended our holiday on the beach on the eastern side of Zanzibar Island in Bjewuu's village. We spent the last four days relaxing, swimming (both in the Indian Ocean and the pool), drinking cocktails, eating locally caught seafood, reading, and walking along the white sandy beaches.

Admittedly, I am relieved that my health has kept up with me so that there was no need to visit any hospital we saw in Tanzania. The piles of plastic rubbish and the enormous potholes in the main roads were a constant reminder that Tanzania is still a third world country.

[288] Our daughter will turn twenty in a couple of weeks, so I suspect she will make her own plans next year. I had my last family holiday when I was nineteen years old.

[289] The relationship between humans and nature has been challenging since the dawn of mankind. Thomas Halliday describes in his book *Otherlands* a scene from the Pliocene, four million years ago, that features many animals, or very similar looking animals, that are still walking around in the Serengeti today. One of the animals that is missing from the Serengeti is *Australopithecus*. *Australopithecus*, the species from which the *Homo*

I wanted to inspire my children to think, reflect, and ask questions about the world we live in. Challenge established ideas in philosophy, science, mathematics...even geology or statistics. I got much pleasure and satisfaction from learning new things and gaining a deeper insight about our environment by asking questions about seemingly trivial matters. Today, I watched a video by Richard Feynman, who was wondering 'why ice is so slippery?' This question immediately brings images to mind of shuffling people trying to walk on ice, or skaters who draw ever tighter circles whilst their spinning speed accelerates. I searched online to find the answer. I found a paper that claimed to have finally solved this question. The authors stated that ice is so slippery because the water molecules at the surface of the ice are loosely bound to the ice and act as "marbles on a dancefloor"[290]. As we are living in an environment where it is not uncommon to experience freezing conditions, living in northern Europe, we are exposed to both ice and water on a regular basis. If the temperature drops significantly, let us say to minus 40 degrees Celsius, ice is not slippery at all – at these temperatures, ice is as rough as sandpaper.

My second thought about holidays is that it bears some resemblance to life; it is so much fun and it's over before you realise that it has started! There is a significant difference. Life is like a holiday with an uncertain end date. Each morning, you must call the reception to determine whether you still have a bed available for the night ahead. At the start of the holiday, you can be fairly confident that you will stay another night, but over time you become increasingly nervous about your sleeping arrangement. You know for a fact that your hotel stay is for a finite period. But you don't know when it ends. During your stay in the hotel, you exchange personal experiences with other guests and use that information to get a sense of the typical length of the holiday. Therefore, one must make careful daily trade-offs as the holiday progresses. Make sure you plan to see the highlights in the first couple of days, whilst at the same time making sure you do not run out of things to do after a week or several months.

The only certainty you have is that you have less than a day left if the person at the reception turns you down for the night. How you will experience this last

---

sapiens, modern man, eventually evolved. During the past roughly 300,000 years, man has transformed Earth, and our impact has been so severe on our planet that in 2000, Crutzen and Stoermer argued that we are currently living in the Anthropocene.

[290] Weber et al., 2018.

day of your vacation is also uncertain. It might be enjoyable till the very end, or it might involve a long, uncomfortable wait for a taxi in the hotel lobby.

Before you realise what is happening, you will be back home, and you will plan your commute to work.

The only thing left at the end of a holiday are memories. Treasure those memories – these moments of happiness and joy. The memories of being back in Tanzania, reliving encounters with wildlife, vistas across the Ngorongoro Crater, getting lost in Stone Town, and the feeling of the beach sand between your toes. A collection of memories is one reason that makes life truly worth living!

On the 21st of August, I will undergo another brain surgery. So, I reckon that August to October will be a bit foggy for me – after the previous operation, it took several months before I regained all my cognitive abilities.

In two days' time, it will be my fifty-third birthday. Before I became ill, I did not give birthday milestones much thought, but now these birthdays seem much more impactful – more important. It not just birthdays – of my children, my wife, my brother, my Mum, and my Dad – today is also fourteen months since the first operation. A month ago, I was told about a growing tumour. Yesterday, I decided that I want another brain surgery, and in three weeks' time, I will, hopefully, wake up after surgery. So much has happened this year…

A personal highlight of this year was the acceptance of the book I have been writing for publication! I received two offers and accepted the offer of the publisher that I would like to get my book in physical bookstores where readers can buy the book for a reasonable price. The book is called Insight, *and it describes how decision analysis helped me cope with my terminal disease.*

Cheers,
Bart

Then I wrote a third letter to my dear friend:

December 20, 2023, Suffolk

Dear Friend,

On the 31st of October I reached my median survival - my P50 – I lived for another 16 months after my diagnosis. In the morning when I reached my median survival, I woke up and got out of my bed; greeted my wife, our son, and the dog; got upstairs and wrote a couple of emails; created a couple of slides and I have been revising my book - nothing out of the ordinary – everything is so bloody normal. Nothing had changed!

A couple of weeks prior to me reaching this milestone I started on a new type of chemotherapy – Lomustine. This is second line treatment, which means that this medication is less effective than the previous treatment. After I had taken the medicine I felt completely fine although I have not slept for a couple of nights, suffered from nausea and have yet to defecated.

Our daughter has been visiting us. She will fly back to Denmark very early on Sunday morning. Our daughter is going to pay a visit to Norway. I came to realise that I am really happy for her – she is enjoying her youth. Young people are such a joy!

The period between 18 and 30 years old was the best time of my life. Once you hit 30 things gradually change – your value system becomes "mature", that is the time when you trade in your zippy car for a family car. By the time you reach your late forties, mid-fifties, you become aware of your own mortality. You can no longer be in denial of your own death.

Earlier this week I cleaned up son's room. The enormous pile of dirty laundry that was lying on the floor was sufficient to fill the washing machine four times. I planned to keep on top of his room to ensure that it stays reasonably clean.

The previous week a met up with a friend of mine and we paid a visit to London – visited some museums, went to see several rock concerts[291] and ate some great food. Because we were in the pub (some things never change) I missed the calls to my mobile phone. Dad was in hospital again. Dad had become dehydrated, felt dizzy and was still in tremendous pain. I flew to the Netherland the next day. I flew to Eindhoven where I met my brother, and we went straight to the hospital to visit Dad. I was shocked how much Dad's health had declined

---

[291] We saw the band "Inhaler".

since the last time we met. He was lying on his back, breathing heavily with both his eyes half closed.

Last time I saw him, he looked much better. Dad, Mum, and I were engaged in several deep conversations. After my Mum left us, I remember telling him that I was not counting on living long enough for the time when the clocks were reset again in the Spring[292]. As this is only six months away, he was really shocked. He was lying on his bed, doing a crossword puzzle – his coping mechanism. He told me that he was happy that I did not tell my Mum. Mum would not let me go home he said…

This time around Mum and I were living together. This time around I did tell my Mum that I don't expect to have a long life. Although Mum contained her emotions, she left the room where I was sitting, and she phoned my sister-in-law and spoke to her emotionally.

A couple of days later Dad appeared grumpy, I am wondering whether he is still in denial of his looming death. He tells me that he felt "too good" to be a patient on the geriatric ward. Despite being 81 years old, and being bound to his bed, he felt that he did not belong on the ward.

I had another seizure on Saturday. This was my second seizure. I "woke up" sitting in my chair being completely oblivious what had just happened to me. I cannot remember a thing from the entire episode. Utterly bizarre. I am really shaken by the whole experience, or more accurately this non-experience…as I have no memory at all from the seizure. I don't know how long I was gone: five seconds, twenty-five seconds, a couple of minutes…I simply do not know…What I do know is that I had wetted myself. I had to go upstairs to get changed into dry clothes. When I came back down again, I noticed that the back cover of the book I was reading before I collapsed and a large fold in the back cover. This fold is the only reminder that I had a seizure.

One of my overriding thoughts was - back to square one – it will take at least a couple of years before I can be back to even contemplate to drive again. Realistically - I might never drive again…

On Monday morning my wife phoned the hospital and explained what had happened over the weekend. Apparently, I was out for five minutes. The doctor recommended to increase the dose in the morning and stick to the same dose in the evening. My wife messaged the doctor and apparently the medication I am taking does increase the risk of seizures.

---

[292] We adjusted the clocks earlier that week.

The following week I stayed off my bike but did go for several walks. The rest of the week went by without any dramatic events, so by Thursday I made up my mind. I had chosen to ignore my doctor's advice and still fly to Copenhagen to visit our daughter. I assume this will be the last trip to Denmark for me, my final trip to lovely Copenhagen.

On Friday afternoon, before we travelled to the airport, I swallowed some pills – I took some steroids and a tablet to safeguard my stomach. On Saturday morning, we left our son in the hotel because he was really tired and met up with our daughter. We met up in a luxury dormitory located next to the building where I had done my Ph.D. many years ago. For old times' sake I did walk over to the building where I was awarded my Ph.D. degree.

We entered café Europa to have a chat and a coffee. After our coffee we met up with our son, who was now recovered, and we explored Copenhagen; we walked into several stores and looked at Copenhagen famous sites. In the evening we met up with some friends who visited us last year, after I send out this message in which I announced I had brain cancer. It really was a lovely evening – it was very nice to see the "next generation" – they are all so mature!

The next morning, we met up with our daughter and walked to Tivoli. Upon entering the park, we bought tickets for rides – and we did do all of them; the free-fall tower, the roller coaster and the two rides where you get shaken violently by going round-and-round. After the rides we were really cold and decided to warm up with pizza and Coke.

Back in the UK, I noticed that I saw double; on the right-hand side I noticed a pulsating, vibrating, trembling movement. I know - I realise - that not all is well in my brain. I have sensations of dizziness, rushing sounds in my ears and a general feeling of light headiness. I must look tired as I notice the comments made by my wife…although it does lie in the lines of expectations that I will get progressively more tired – so it could well be a biased assessment. Overall, I am inclined to make a positive self-assessment, i.e., I believe that there is a larger probability that the tumour has progressed than that it has not progressed. In my assessment on the probability whether the tumour has progressed beyond the brain is 35% (35% is the medium estimate; P90 is 75%, the P10 is 8%). After I finished lunch, I recovered and took Archie for a walk. I recovered in the fresh winter weather helped me to recover. After two hours I returned home and felt fine again…

On Wednesday the 13th of December I was presented with an R&D award[293]. The prize was given at the end of the ceremony so we could learn "what not to do". So do not freeze once you're in the spotlight and resist the temptation to rub your eyes whilst on camara. My team members and I received the award with a short film featuring our project sponsor telling nice things about our achievements and the impact we made to the business.

Cheers,
Bart

Still waiting for a cure

It is undeniable that progress in Overall Survival has been made. For example, a study of survival trends for brain tumour patients[294] found that the median survival improved from 13 to 26 months for patients diagnosed in the 1970s compared with patients diagnosed in 2010s[295]. For patients diagnosed with glioblastoma, significant advances in survival have come from the implementation of the Stupp protocol, a combination of radiation and Temozolomide (TMZ) treatment, which saw significant increases in 2-year survival and is now considered standard of care[296]. Other improvements include the use of an optical imaging agent called Gleolan™ to help visualize tumour cells during surgery[297] and increased accuracy of the delivery of radiation therapy. But truth to be told, TMZ was approved for clinical use in 1999, yet 64 new treatments have been approved for blood cancers and 15 for breast cancer[298].

---

[293] I actually won a second award. Our department ended up with three awards. This total of three awards was the total of R&D awards won in the competition by Data Science and Artificial Intelligence!

[294] These patients were elderly individuals with primary central nervous system lymphomas.

[295] Mendez et al., 2018.

[296] Johnson and O'Neill, 2012.

[297] https://utswmed.org/medblog/glowing-tumors-how-fluorescence-helps-neurosurgeons-fight-brain-cancer/#:~:text='Gleolan%20(aminolevulinic%20acid%20hydrochloride).'

[298] https://braintumourresearch.org/blogs/research-campaigning-news/the-high-price-of-brain-tumours

Fifteen months have passed since I was told about my brain tumour and it has been a year since the surgeons removed the tumour. The hole they left after the operation has slowly been shrinking ever since. I know that the surgeon will have left some parts of the tumour behind, and I also know that the chemotherapy and radiation treatments have slowed down their growth. I remember meeting my doctor for the first time and that he talked about "stunning the tumour" and "we will get you through the first six months". I am still facing a dire outlook – after 5 years, only 1 in 17, or 5.5%, of patients who have been diagnosed with glioblastoma will be alive.

John Gunther Jr. died on June 30, 1947. John was seventeen years old when he died from an aggressive brain tumour. John's illness lasted for fifteen months. John's parents hoped for a cure until the bitter end – the death of their son. Three quarters of a century later, I was told that I had sixteen months to live. Clearly, we are two different individuals, but I am as desperate for a cure as John was 75 years ago[299].

Concluding remarks: Afterword

Notwithstanding the chilling facts surrounding death, I am an optimist. To quote Margaret Heffernan in her book *Unchartered*: 'Optimists do better in life – live longer, healthier, more successful lives – for the simple reason that they don't give up easily' and '[Optimists] realise that the only way to know the future is to make it.' An optimist can also be a realist. At the time I received my diagnosis, I knew that the odds of surviving for another two years were negligible indeed.

Over time, my mood has reverted to baseline happiness. My sleep pattern has improved. I am no longer lying in bed wide awake during the early mornings. I can live in the moment – no matter what tomorrow brings. I have also put my life in order. I can answer the question raised by Jordan Peterson in his book *12 Rules for Life*: Have you cleaned up your life? With a resounding 'Yes.' I have no regrets. I have always done what I wanted to do and have been very conscious about not hurting anybody physically nor mentally. I have made conscious choices about what I want to achieve in life. Carefully considered the trade-offs

---

[299] In addition to suffering from the same disease, John and I also shared an interest in geology!

and did my best to make good judgements, realising that there is no point investing much energy in looking more than two to three years ahead.

I would like to end with a quote from the self-confessed optimist Stephen Hawking, who was diagnosed with amyotrophic lateral sclerosis (ALS) in his early 20s and lived for another 50 years defying all odds: '...however difficult life may seem, there is always something you can do and succeed at. It matters that you don't give up. Unleash your imagination. Shape the future.'

References

Adelson, E.H. (2005) "Checker shadow Illusion". Perceptual Science Group. MIT.

Angel, M. (2004) The truth about the drug companies. Random House. ISBN: 0375508465.

Ariely, D., Loewenstein, G. and Prelec, D. (2003) "Coherent Arbitrariness": Stable Demand Curves without Stable Preferences. Quarterly Journal of Economics, 118: 73–105. DOI: 10.1162/00335530360535153.

Altman D. G. (1998) Confidence intervals for the number needed to treat. BMJ (Clinical research ed.), 317(7168), 1309–1312. https://doi.org/10.1136/bmj.317.7168.1309.

Baar, J. and Tannock, I. (1989) Analyzing the same data in two ways: a demonstration model to illustrate the reporting and misreporting of clinical trials. Journal of clinical oncology: official journal of the American Society of Clinical Oncology, 7(7), 969–978. DOI: 10.1200/JCO.1989.7.7.969.

Balana, C., Vaz, M. A., Sepúlveda, J. M., Mesia, C., del Barco, S., Pineda, E., Muñoz-Langa, J., Estival, A., de las Peñas, R., Fuster, J. Gironés, R., Navarro, L. M., Gil-Gil, M., Alonso, M., Herrero, A.., Peralta, S., Olier, C., Perez-Segura, P., Covela, M., Martinez-García, M., Berrocal, A., Gallego, O., Luque, R., Perez-Martín, F. J., Esteve, A., Munne, N., Domenech, M., Villa, S., Sanz, C. and Carrato, C. (2020) A phase II randomized, multicenter, open-label trial of continuing adjuvant temozolomide beyond 6 cycles in patients with glioblastoma (GEINO 14-01) Neuro-Oncology 22(12), 1851–1861, DOI: 10.1093/neuonc/noaa107.

Barraclough, H., Simms, L. and Govindan R. (2011) Biostatistics Primer: What a Clinician Ought to Know: Hazard Ratios Journal of Thoracic Oncology Volume 6, Issue 6, Pages 978–982. DOI: 10.1097/JTO.0b013e31821b10ab.

Bratvold, R.B. and Begg, S.H. (2010) Making Good Decisions. Society of Petroleum Engineers. ISBN: 9781555632588.

Bregman R. (2019) De meeste mensen deugen (Humankind - A Hopeful History) de Correspondent. ISBN: 9789082942187

Brey, R. and Pinto Prades, J. (2017) Age effects in mortality risk valuation. The European Journal of Health Economics. 18. DOI:10.1007/s10198-016-0852-8.

Brown, T. (2023) Creative Leadership in Times of Uncertainty https://www.youtube.com/watch?v=YNVM69FcKhA Latest accessed in May 2023.

Burkeman, O. (2021) Four Thousand Weeks, time management for mortals. Penguin Random House. ISBN: 9781784704001.

Butler, M., Pongor, L., Su, Y.T., Xi, L., Raffeld, M., Quezado, M., Trepel, J., Aldape, K., Pommier, Y., and Wu, J. (2020) MGMT Status as a Clinical Biomarker in Glioblastoma. Trends Cancer 6(5):380–391.
DOI: 10.1016/j.trecan.2020.02.010.

Cioffi, G., Waite, K.A., Edelson, J.L. et al. (2022) Changes in survival over time for primary brain and other CNS tumors in the United States, 2004–2017. J Neurooncol 160, 209–219. DOI:10.1007/s11060-022-04138-w.

Clemen, R.T. and Reilly, T. (2001) Making hard decisions. Pacific Grove, California, USA: Duxbury. ISBN: 0534421997.

Clukey, L. (2008) Anticipatory mourning: processes of expected loss in palliative care. International Journal of Palliative Nursing, 14(7), 316–325.
DOI:10.12968/ijpn.2008.14.7.30617.

Colloca, L. (2018) The Placebo Effect in Pain Therapies. Annual Review of Pharmacology and Toxicology, 59, 191-211. DOI: 10.1146/annurev-pharmtox-010818-021542

Cokkinides, V.E., Chao, A., Smith, R.A., Vernon, S.W. and Thun, M.J. (2003) Correlates of underutilization of colorectal cancer screening among U.S. adults, age 50 years and older. Prev Med. 2003;36(1):85–91. DOI:10.1006/pmed.2002.1127.

Csikszentmihalyi, M. (1990) Flow: the psychology of optimal experience. Harper & Row. ISBN: 9780060162535.

Crutzen, P. and Stoermer, E. (2013) "The 'Anthropocene'" (2000). In L. Robin, S. Sörlin & P. Warde (Ed.), The Future of Nature: Documents of Global Change (pp. 479–490). New Haven: Yale University Press. https://doi.org/10.12987/9780300188479-041.

Detering, K., Hancock, A., Reade, M. and Silvester, W. (2010) The impact of advance care planning on end of life care in elderly patients: randomised controlled trial. BMJ, 340. DOI: 10.1136/bmj.c1345.

de Price, K. (1966) Diary of Nicholas II, 1917–1918, an annotated translation. The University of Montana https://scholarworks.umt.edu/cgi/viewcontent.cgi?article=3084&context=etd#:~:text=Nicholas%20II%20kept%20a%20diary,Journal%20Intime%20de%20Nicolas%20II.

Diaconis, P. (2003) The problem of thinking too much. Technical Report No. 2003-3. Department of Statistics, Stanford University, Stanford, California 94305-4065 http://www-stat.stanford.edu

Diaconis, P., Holmes, S. and Montgomery, R. (2007) Dynamical Bias in the Coin Toss. SIAM REVIEW, 49, No. 2, 211–235, DOI: 10.1137/S0036144504446436.

Didion, J. (2005) The year of magical thinking. Alfred A. Knopf publishers a division of Random House. ISBN: 140004314X

Dong, X. et al. (2016) Survival trends of grade I, II and III astrocytoma patients and associated clinical practice patterns between 1999 and 2010: A SEER-based analysis, Neuro-Oncology Practice 3, 29–38, DOI: 10.1093/nop/npv016.

Doubilet, P., Weinstein, M.C. and McNeil, B.J. (1986) Use and misuse of the term "cost effective" in medicine. N Engl J Med. 314(4):253–6. DOI: 10.1056/NEJM198601233140421.

Duke, A. (2020) How to decide. Simple tools for making better choices. Portfolio, Penguin. ISBN: 9780593418482.

Edwards, W. (1983) Human cognitive capacities, representativeness and ground rules for research. In P. Humphreys, O. Svenson, & A. Vari (Eds.), Analyzing and aiding decision processes, 507–513, Akademiai Kiado.

Fuller, S. (2005) The Intellectual. Icon Books. ISBN 9781840467215.

Freud, Sigmund (1917) Trauer und Melancholie. Internationale Zeitschrift für Ärztliche Psychoanalyse [International Journal for Medical Psychoanalysis]. 4 (6): 288–301.

Fulton, R. (2003) Anticipatory mourning: A critique of the concept. Mortality, 8(4), 342–351. DOI: 10.1080/13576270310001613392.

Gade, G., Venohr, I., Conner, D., McGrady, K., Beane, J., Richardson, R., Williams, M.P., Liberson, M., Blum, M. and Della Penna, R. (2008) Impact of an inpatient palliative care team: a randomized control trial. Journal of Palliative Medicine, 11(2), 180–90. DOI: 10.1089/jpm.2007.0055.

Gallup, G. (1996). Religion in America. Will the Vitality of the Church Be the Surprise of the 21st Century? Princeton Religion Research Center, ISBN: 9996302903

Gandjour, A. (2020) Willingness to pay for new medicines: a step towards narrowing the gap between NICE and IQWiG. BMC Health Serv Res 20, 343. DOI: 10.1186/s12913-020-5050-9.

Gawande, A. (2014) Being Mortal. Profile books, London, UK.
ISBN: 9781846685828.

Gerber, I., Rusalem, R., Harmon, N., Battin, D. and Arkin, A. (1975)
Anticipatory grief and aged widows and widowers. Journal of Gerontology,
30(2), 225–229. DOI: 10.1093/geronj/30.2.225.

Gigerenzer, G. (2003) Reckoning with Risk: Learning to Live with Uncertainty.
Penguin, Random House, UK. ISBN: 0140297863.

Gigerenzer, G. (2008) Gut Feelings: Short Cuts to Better Decision Making.
Penguin, Random House, UK. ISBN: 0141015918.

Goodwin, P. and Wright, G. (2004) Decision analysis for management judgment.
Fourth edition. John Wiley & Sons, Ltd. ISBN: 9780470714393.

Gordis L. (2008) Epidemiology. 4th ed. Philadelphia: Saunders
ISBN: 9781416040026.

Gould, S.J. (1996) Dinosaurs in a Haystack. Jonathan Cape Random House,
London, UK. ISBN 0224044729.

Grajnek, L. (2010) Grief as pathology: The evolution of grief theory in
psychology from Freud to the present. History of Psychology, 13(1), 46–73.
DOI: 10.1037/a0016991.

Grassi, L. (2007) Bereavement in families with relatives dying of cancer. Current
Opinion in Supportive and Palliative Care, 1(1), 43–49.
DOI: 10.1097/SPC.0b013e32813a3276.

Gray, P. (2013) The play deficit. Aeon.

Grieve, A. P. (2003) The number needed to treat: a useful clinical measure or a
case of the Emperor's new clothes? Pharmaceutical Statistics 2(2):87–102. DOI:
10.1002/pst.033.

Grosse S. D. (2008). Assessing cost-effectiveness in healthcare: history of the $50,000 per QALY threshold. Expert review of pharmacoeconomics & outcomes research, 8(2), 165–178. https://doi.org/10.1586/14737167.8.2.165

Gusev, Y., Bhuvaneshwar, K., Song, L. *et al.* (2018) The REMBRANDT study, a large collection of genomic data from brain cancer patients. *Sci Data* **5**, 180158. https://doi.org/10.1038/sdata.2018.158.

Hamlin, R. P. (2017) The gaze heuristic: Biography of an adaptively rational decision process. Topics in Cognitive Science,9(2), 264–288. DOI: 10.1111/tops.12253.

Hammond, J.S., Keeney, R.L. and Raiffa H. (1999) Smart choices. A practical guide to making better decisions. Havard Business School Press. Boston, Massachusetts, USA. IBSN: 9781633691049.

Harari, Y.N. (2011) Sapiens: A Brief History of Humankind. Penguin, Random House, UK. ISBN: 9780099590088.

Harari, Y.N. (2011) 21 Lessons for 21st Century. Penguin, Random House, UK. ISBN: 9781784708283.

Hegi, M. E., Diserens, A. C, Gorlia, T., Hamou, M. F., de Tribolet, N., Weller, M., Kros, J. M., Hainfellner, J. A., Mason, W., Mariani, L., Bromberg, J.E.C., Hau, P. et al. (2005) MGMT Gene Silencing and Benefit from Temozolomide in Glioblastoma. N Engl J Med; 352:997–1003. DOI: 10.1056/NEJMoa043331

Hoffrage, U., Lindsey, S., Hertwig, R. and Gigerenzer, G. (2000) Communicating Statistical Information. Science, 290, 2261–2262.
DOI: 10.1126/science.290.5500.2261.

Hora, S. C. (2007) Eliciting probabilities from experts. In W. Edwards, R. F. Miles, Jr., & D. von Winterfeldt (Eds.), Advances in decision analysis: From foundations to applications (pp. 129–153). Cambridge University Press. DOI: 10.1017/CBO9780511611308.009.

Howard, R.A. (1989) Knowledge Maps. Management Science 35, 903–922. DOI: 10.1287/mnsc.35.8.903.

Howard, R.A. (1990) From influence to relevance to knowledge. In Influence diagrams belief net and Decision Analysis. Ed R.M. Oliver and J.Q. Smith, 3–23, New York city, John Wiley & sons. ISBN: 9780471923817.

Iny, A. and de Brabandere, L. (2010) Rethinking Scenarios, What a Difference a Day Makes.
https://www.bcg.com/publications/2010/strategy-rethinking-scenarios-what-difference-day-makes

Ivancovich, D. A. (2004) The Role of Existential Coping and Spiritual Coping in Anticipatory Grief (Master Thesis), Trinity Western University, Langley City, Canada.

Kaplan, E.L. and Meier, P. (1958) Nonparametric estimation from incomplete observations. J Am Stat Assoc 53:457–481.
DOI: 10.1080/01621459.1958.10501452.

Johnson, D.R. and O'Neill, B.P. (2012) Glioblastoma survival in the United States before and during the temozolomide era. J Neurooncol 107(2):359–364. DOI:10.1007/s11060-011-0749-4.

Jones, S.R., Carley, S., Harrison, M. (2003) An introduction to power and sample size estimation. Emergency Medicine Journal 20, 453–458.
DOI: 10.1136/emj.20.5.453.

Kahneman, D. and Tversky, A. (1973) On the psychology of prediction. Psychological Review, 80(4), 237–251. DOI:10.1037/h0034747.

Kahneman, D. (2012) Thinking, Fast and Slow. ISBN: 0141033576.

Keeney, R.L. (1992) Value Focussed Thinking. Harvard university press, Cambridge, Massachusetts. ISBN 0674931971.

Kehl, K. A. (2005) Recognition and support of anticipatory mourning. Journal of Hospice and Palliative Nursing, 7(4), 206–211. DOI: 10.1097/00129191-200507000-00011.

Kelley, K. and Kelley, D. (2014) Creative Confidence. HarperCollins Publishers, Dublin, Ireland. ISBN 9780385349376.

Khanolkar, A. R., Ljung, R., Talbäck, M., Brooke, H. L., Carlsson, S., Mathiesen, T. and Feychting, M. (2016) Socioeconomic position and the risk of brain tumour: a Swedish national population-based cohort study. Journal of epidemiology and community health, 70(12), 1222–1228. DOI: 10.1136/jech-2015-207002.

Kübler-Ross, E. (1969) On death and dying. New York, NY: Routledge.

Lee J. (1994) Odds ratio or relative risk for cross-sectional data? International journal of epidemiology, 23(1), 201–203. DOI: 10.1093/ije/23.1.201.

Lindemann, E. (1944) Symptomatology and management of acute grief. American Journal of Psychiatry, 101(2), 141–148. DOI: 10.1176/ajp.151.6.155.

Lorenz, E.N. (1995) The Essence of Chaos. Seattle: University of Washington Press. ISBN: 9780295975146.

Land, G. and Jarman B. (1992) Breakpoint and Beyond: Mastering the Future Today. Harpercollins Publishers. ISBN: 9780962660528.

Lejarraga, T. and Hertwig, R. (2021) How experimental methods shaped views on human competence and rationality. Psychological Bulletin, 147(6), 535–564. DOI:10.1037/bul0000324.

Li, S. Q., Pan, X. F., Kashaf, M. S., Xue, Q. P., Luo, H. J., Wang, Y. Y., Wen, Y. and Yang, C.hX. (2017) Five-Year Survival is Not a Useful Measure for Cancer Control in the Population: an Analysis Based on UK Data. Asian Pacific journal of cancer prevention: APJCP, 18(2), 571–576. DOI:10.22034/APJCP.2017.18.2.571.

Libet, B. (1985) Unconscious cerebral initiative and the role of conscious will in voluntary action. The behavioral and brain sciences 8, 529–566. DOI:10.1017/S0140525X00044903.

Lichtenstein, S., Fischhoff, B. and Philips, L.D. (1982) Calibration of probabilities: The state of the art to 1980. In judgment under uncertainty: Heuristics and biases, ed. D. Kahneman, P. Slovic and A. Tversky. Cambridge, UK: Cambridge University Press. ISBN: 9780511809477.

Malmström, A., Henning Grønberg, B., Marosi, C., Stupp, R., Frappaz, D., Schultz, H., et al. (2012) Temozolomide versus standard 6-week radiotherapy versus hypofractionated radiotherapy in patients older than 60 years with glioblastoma: the Nordic randomised, phase 3 trial. 13, 9, 916–926. DOI: 10.1016/S1470-2045(12)70265-6.

Maslow A. H. (1943) A Theory of Human Motivation. Psychological Review, 50, 370–396.

Mendez J.S., Ostrom Q.T., Gittleman H., Kruchko C., Deangelis L.M., Barnholtz-Sloan J.S. and Grommes C. (2018) The elderly left behind—changes in survival trends of primary central nervous system lymphoma over the past 4 decades. Neurooncology 20(5):687–694. DOI: 10.1093/neuonc/nox187.

Moreau, C. P. and Engeset, M. G. (2016) The Downstream Consequences of Problem-Solving Mindsets: How Playing with LEGO Influences Creativity. Journal of Marketing Research, 53(1), 18–30. DOI:10.1509/jmr.13.0499.

Murray, D. B., & Teare, S. W. (1993). Probability of a tossed coin landing on edge. Physical review. E, Statistical physics, plasmas, fluids, and related interdisciplinary topics, 48(4), 2547–2552. https://doi.org/10.1103/physreve.48.2547

Suárez, M (2021) Philosophy of Probability and Statistical Modelling. Cambridge University Press. ISBN 9781108984942.

McCabe, C., Claxton, K. and Culyer, A.J. (2008) The NICE cost-effectiveness threshold: what it is and what that means. Pharmacoeconomics. 26(9), 733–44. DOI: 10.2165/00019053-200826090-00004.

McLane, M., Gouveia, J., Citron, G.P., MacKay, J. and Rose, P.R. (2008) Responsible reporting of uncertain petroleum reserves. AAPG Bulletin 92 (10): 1431–1452. DOI:10.1306/06040808075.

McNamee, P. and Celona, J. (2005) Decision analysis for the professional. Fourth edition. Menlo Park, California, USA, SmartOrg. ISBN: 0971056900.

Miller, G.A. (1956) The magical number seven, plus or minus two: Some limits on our capacity for processing information. Psychological Review. 63 (2), 81–97. DOI: 10.1037/h0043158.

Minniti, G., De Sanctis, V., Muni, R., Rasio, D., Lanzetta, G., Bozzao, A., Osti, M. F., Salvati, M., Valeriani, M., Cantore, G. P. and Maurizi Enrici. R. (2009) Hypofractionated radiotherapy followed by adjuvant chemotherapy with temozolomide in elderly patients with glioblastoma. J Neurooncol 91, 95–100. DOI: 10.1007/s11060-008-9689-z.

Molloy, W.D., Guyatt, G.H, Russo, R., Goeree, R., O'Brien, B.J., Bédard, M., Willan, A., Watson, J., Patterson, C., Harrison, C., Standish, T., Strang, D., Darzins, P.J., Smith, S. and Dubois, S. (2000). Systematic implementation of an advance directive program in nursing homes: a randomized controlled trial. JAMA, 283(11), 1437–44. DOI: 10.1001/jama.283.11.1437.

Moore, D.A. and Healy, P.J. (2008) The trouble with overconfidence. Psychological Review 115 (2): 502–517. DOI: 10.1037/0033-295X.115.2.502.

Nau, R.F. (2001) De Finetti was Right: Probability Does Not Exist. Theory and Decision 51, 89–124. DOI: 10.1023/A:1015525808214.

Nielsen M.K., Neergaard, M.A., Jensen, A.B., Bro, F. and Guldin, M.B. (2016) Do we need to change our understanding of anticipatory grief in caregivers? A systematic review of caregiver studies during end-of-life caregiving and bereavement. Clin Psychol Rev 44:75–93. DOI: 10.1016/j.cpr.2016.01.002.

Nisbet, M.C. (2009) Framing Science: A New Paradigm in Public Engagement. New Agendas in Science Communication, Kahlor, Land Stout, P. (Eds). Taylor & Francis Publishers. ISBN 9780415999595.

Nisbet, M.C. and Goidel, K. (2007) Understanding citizen perceptions of science controversy: Bridging the ethnographic-survey research divide. Public Understanding of Science, 16, 4, 421–440. DOI: 10.1177/0963662506065558.

Orford, N.R., Milnes, S., Simpson, N., Keely, G., Elderkin, T., Bone, A., Martin, P., Bellomo, R., Bailey, M. and Corke, C. (2019) Effect of communication skills training on outcomes in critically ill patients with life-limiting illness referred for intensive care management: a before-and-after study. BMJ Support Palliat Care. 9(1), 21. DOI: 10.1136/bmjspcare-2016-001231.

Osborn, A.F. (1963) Applied Imagination: Principles and Procedures of Creative Problem-Solving. Published by Charles Scribner's Sons, 3rd revision.

Owens, D. K., Shachter, R. D. and Nease, R. F., Jr (1997) Representation and analysis of medical decision problems with influence diagra Medical decision-making : an international journal of the Society for Medical Decision-making, 17(3), 241–262. DOI: 10.1177/0272989X9701700301.

Patel, M.S., Volpp, K.G., Small, D.S. (2016) Using active choice within the electronic health record to increase physician ordering and patient completion of high-value cancer screening tests. Healthc (Amst). 4(4), 340–345. DOI: 10.1016/j.hjdsi.2016.04.005.

Patel, M.S., Volpp, K.G. and Asch, D.A. (2018) Nudge units to improve the delivery of health care. N Engl J Med. 378.
DOI:10.1001/jamanetworkopen.2018.0818.

Paulos, J.A. (1988) Innumeracy. Farrar, Strauss & Giroux, New York. ISBN: 0809074478.

Penrod, J., Hupcey, J.E., Baney, B.L. and Loeb, S.J. (2011) End-of-life caregiving trajectories. Clinical Nursing Research, 20(1), 7–24. DOI:10.1177/1054773810384852.

Perry, J. R., Laperriere, N., O'Callaghan, C. J., Brandes, A. A., Menten, J., Phillips, C., Fay, M., Nishikawa, R., Cairncross, J. G., Roa, W., Osoba, D., Rossiter, J. P., Sahgal, A., Hirte, H., Laigle-Donadey, F., Franceschi, E., Chinot, O., Golfinopoulos, V., Fariselli, L., Wick, A., Feuvret, L., Back, M., Tills, M., Winch, C., Baumert, B. G., Wick, W., Ding, K., Mason, W. P. (2017) Short-Course Radiation plus Temozolomide in Elderly Patients with Glioblastoma. N Engl J Med. 1027–1037, 376, 11, DOI: 10.1056/NEJMoa1611977.

Peterson, C. R. and Beach, L. R. (1967) Man as an intuitive statistician. Psychological Bulletin,68(1), 29–46. DOI: 10.1037/h0024722.

Pocock, S.J. and Stone, G.W. (2016) The Primary Outcome Is Positive—Is That Good Enough? N Engl J Med 375, 971–979. DOI: 10.1056/NEJMra1601511.

Plous, S. (1993) The psychology of judgment and decision-making. McGraw-Hill series in social psychology. ISBN: 0070504776.

Prior, M. (2005) News v. Entertainment: How Increasing Media Choice Widens Gaps in Political Knowledge and Turnout. American Journal of Political Science, 49, 577, 2005. DOI: 10.2307/3647733.

Rabow, M., Dibble, S., Pantilat, S. and McPhee, S. (2004) The comprehensive care team: a controlled trial of outpatient palliative medicine consultation. Archives of Internal Medicine, 164(1), 83–91. DOI: 10.1001/archinte.164.1.83.

Rees, W. D., & Lutkins, S. G. (1967) Mortality of bereavement. British medical journal, 4(5570), 13–16. DOI:10.1136/bmj.4.5570.13

Roa, W., Brasher, P.M.A., Bauman, G., Anthes, M., Bruera, E., Chan, A., Fisher, B., Fulton, D., Gulavita, S., Hao, C., Husain, S., Murtha, A., Petruk, K., Stewart, D., Tai, P., Urtasun, R., Cairncross, J.G. and Forsyth, P. (2004) Abbreviated Course of Radiation Therapy in Older Patients With Glioblastoma Multiforme:

A Prospective Randomized Clinical Trial. Journal of Clinical Oncology 22:9, 1583–1588. DOI: 10.1200/JCO.2004.06.082.

Roa, W., Kepka, L., Kumar, N., Sinaika, V., Matiello, J., Hentati, D.L.D., de Castro, D. G., Dyttus-Cebulok, K., Drodge, S., Ghosh, S., Jeremić, B., Rosenblatt, E. and Fidarova, E. (2015) International Atomic Energy Agency Randomized Phase III Study of Radiation Therapy in Elderly and/or Frail Patients With Newly Diagnosed Glioblastoma Multiforme. Journal of Clinical Oncology 33, 35, 4145–4150. DOI: 10.1200/JCO.2015.62.6606.

Rogalla, K. B. (2015) Examining Relationships between Proactive Coping and Experiences of Personal and Posttraumatic Growth during Anticipatory Grief (Doctoral dissertation). University Of Northern Colorado, Greeley, Colorado.

Rosling, H., Rosling, O. and Rosling-Rohnnlund A. (2018) Factfulness. Sceptre, Hodder & Stoughton Ltd., Carmelit House, London, UK. ISBN: 147363749X.

Saldinger, A. and Cain, A. C. (2005) Deromanticizing anticipated death: Denial, disbelief and disconnection in bereaved spouses. Journal of Psychosocial Oncology, 22(3), 69–92. DOI: 10.1300/J077v22n03_04.

Schulz, R., Hebert, R., & Boerner, K. (2008) Bereavement after caregiving. Geriatrics, 63(1), 20–22.

Schoemaker, P.J.H. (1995) Scenario planning: A tool for strategic thinking. MIT Sloan Management Review 36, 25–40.

Shapiro, S.M. (2001) 24/7 Innovation: A Blueprint for Surviving and Thriving in an Age of Change, McGraw-Hill Companies. ISBN: 0071376267.
Simon, H.A. (1945) Administrative behavior: A study of decision-making processes in administrative organizations. The free press, New York, US. ISBN: 0684835827.

Soon, C., Brass, M., Heinze, H.J. et al. (2008) Unconscious determinants of free decisions in the human brain. Nat Neurosci 11, 543–545. DOI: 10.1038/nn.2112.

Spichiger, E. (2008) Living with terminal illness: patient and family experiences of hospital end-of-life care. International Journal of Palliative Nursing, 14(5), 220–228. DOI:10.12968/ijpn.2008.14.5.29489.

Spotswood, S., Reid, J.E., Grace, M. and Samore, M. (2004) Hazard Ratio in Clinical Trials. Antimicrobial Agents and Chemotherapy. 48 (8): 2787–2792. DOI:10.1128/AAC.48.8.2787-2792.2004.

Stupp, R., Mason, W.P., van den Bent, M.J., Weller, M., Fisher, B., Taphoorn, M.J.B., Belanger, K., Brandes, A.A., Marosi, C., Bogdahn, U., Curschmann, J., Janzer, R.C., et al. (2005) Radiotherapy plus Concomitant and Adjuvant Temozolomide for Glioblastoma. N Engl J Med. 352:987–996. DOI: 10.1056/NEJMoa043330.

Stupp, R., Hegi, M.E., Mason, W.P., van den Bent. Ma. J., Taphoorn, M.J.B., Janzer, R.C., Ludwin, S.K., Allgeier, A., Fisher, B., Belanger, K., Hau, P., Brandes, A.A., Gijtenbeek, J., Marosi, C., Vecht, C.J., Mokhtari, K., Wesseling, P., Villa, S., Eisenhauer, E., Gorlia, T. and Mirimanoff, R.O. (2009) Effects of radiotherapy with concomitant and adjuvant temozolomide versus radiotherapy alone on survival in glioblastoma in a randomised phase III study: 5-year analysis of the EORTC-NCIC trial The Lancet Oncology 10, 5, 459–466. DOI: 10.1016/S1470-2045(09)70025-7.

Sweeting, H. N. and Gilhooly, M. L. (1990) Anticipatory grief: A review. Social Science and Medicine, 30(10), 1073–1080. DOI: 10.1016/0277-9536(90)90293.

Tegmark, M. (2014) Our Mathematical Universe. Penguin, Random House, UK. ISBN: 9780241954638.

Tegmark, M. (2017) Life 3.0. Penguin, Random House, UK. ISBN: 9780141981802.

Tengs, T.O., Adams, M.E., Pliskin, J.S., Safran, D.G., Siegel, J.E., Weinstein, M.C. and Graham, J.D. (1995) Five-Hundred Life-Saving Interventions and Their Cost-Effectiveness. Risk Analysis, 15: 369–390. DOI: 10.1111/j.1539-6924.1995.tb00330.x.

Tseng, J., Poppenk, J. (2020) Brain meta-state transitions demarcate thoughts across task contexts exposing the mental noise of trait neuroticism. Nat Commun 11, 3480. DOI: 10.1038/s41467-020-17255-9.

Tversky, A. and Kahneman, D. (1971) Belief in the law of small numbers. Psychological Bulletin 76, No. 2, 105–110. DOI: 10.1037/h0031322.

Tversky, A., & Kahneman, D. (1982). Judgments of and by representativeness. In D. Kahneman, P. Slovic, & A. Tversky (Eds.), Judgment under Uncertainty: Heuristics and Biases (pp. 84-98). Cambridge: Cambridge University Press. doi:10.1017/CBO9780511809477.007

Tversky, A. and Kahneman, D. (1974) Judgment under uncertainty: Heuristics and biases. Science, 185(4157), 1124–1131.
DOI: 10.1126/science.185.4157.1124.

Ünal, E. (2019) An interpretative phenomenological analysis of anticipatory grief: Getting stuck between the problems of the present and the future. https://acikbilim.yok.gov.tr/handle/20.500.12812/678982.

Volkan, V. D. and Zintl, E. (1993) Life After Loss: The Lessons of Grief. Charles Scribner's Sons. DOI: 0684195747.

Wald, N. J. and Morris, J. K. (2020) Two under-recognized limitations of number needed to treat, International Journal of Epidemiology, 49(2), 359–360. DOI: 10.1093/ije/dyz267.

Weber, B., Nagata, Y., Ketzetzi, S., Tang, F., Smit, W. J., Bakker, H. J., Backus, E. H. G., Bonn, M. and Bonn, D. (2018) Molecular Insight into the Slipperiness of Ice. The Journal of Physical Chemistry Letters 9, 2838–2842. DOI: 10.1021/acs.jpclett.8b01188.

Wegwarth, O., Gaissmaier, W. and Gigerenzer, G. (2011) Deceiving Numbers: Survival Rates and Their Impact on Doctors' Risk Communication. Medical Decision-making. 31(3), 386–394. DOI:10.1177/0272989X10391469.

Welch, H. G., Schwartz, L. M. and Woloshin, S. (2000) Are increasing 5-year survival rates evidence of success against cancer? JAMA, 283(22), 2975–2978. DOI: 10.1001/jama.283.22.2975.

White, A., Thompson, T.D. and White, M.C. (2015) Cancer screening test use—United States. MMWR Morb Mortal Wkly Rep. 2017, 66(8), 201–206. DOI: 10.15585/mmwr.mm6608a1.

Wilt, T.J., Harris, R.P. and Qaseem, A. (2015) High Value Care Task Force of the American College of Physicians. Screening for cancer: advice for high-value care from the American College of Physicians. Ann Intern Med. 162(10), 718–725. DOI: 10.7326/M14-2326.

Yong, A.S.J., Lim, Y.H., Cheong, M.W.L., Hamzah, E. and Teoh, S.L. (2022) Willingness-to-pay for cancer treatment and outcome: a systematic review. Eur J Health Econ. Aug;23(6):1037–1057. DOI: 10.1007/s10198-021-01407-9.

Young, M., Benjamin, B., & Wallis, C. (1963) The mortality of widowers. Lancet (London, England), 2(7305), 454–456. DOI:10.1016/s0140-6736(63)92193-7

Zhang, M., Xu, F., Ni, W., Qi, W., Cao, W., Xu, C., Jhen, J. and Gao, Y. (2020) Survival impact of delaying postoperative chemoradiotherapy in newly-diagnosed glioblastoma patients. Transl Cancer Res. 9(9): 5450–5458. DOI: 10.21037/tcr-20-1718.

Zilberfein, F. (1999) Coping with death: Anticipatory grief and bereavement. Generations, 23(1), 69–74.

Zur, I., Tzuk-Shina, T., Guriel, M., Eran, A. and Kaidar-Person, O. (2020) Survival impact of the time gap between surgery and chemo-radiotherapy in Glioblastoma patients. Sci Rep 12, 10(1), 9595. DOI: 10.1038/s41598-020-66608-3.

Index

Printed in Great Britain
by Amazon

43400130R00196